NOURISHING LITTLE ONES: THE FIRST BITES

A COMPREHENSIVE GUIDE TO COMPLEMENTARY FEEDING AND RECIPE IDEAS FOR 6 MONTHS TO 2 YEARS CHILDREN

A HANDBOOK FOR PEDIATRICIANS, PARENTS AND DIETICIANS

DR. KALYANI PATRA

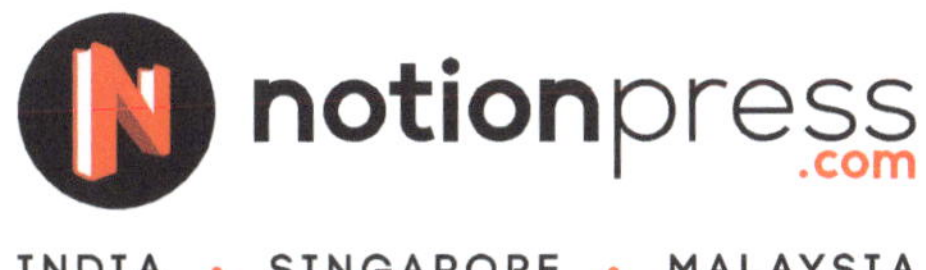

Copyright © Dr. Kalyani Patra 2024
All Rights Reserved.

ISBN
Hardcase 979-8-89544-273-9
Paperback 979-8-89498-863-4

Contents

Foreword 5

Preface 9

Chapter 1   Introduction 13

Chapter 2   What is Complementary Feeding? 17

Chapter 3   The Joy of Feeding Your Little One 23

Chapter 4   Understanding Your Child's Nutritional Needs 27

Chapter 5   Hygiene Measures 33

Chapter 6   Recommendations on Sugar and Salt 37

Chapter 7   The Correct Use and Importance of
            Oil and Ghee 41

Chapter 8   Spice Recommendations 49

Chapter 9   Guide for Water Intake 55

Chapter 10 Common Challenges and Solutions 59

Chapter 11 Understanding Food Allergies 65

Chapter 12 Unhealthy Diet and Beverages 71

Chapter 13 Tiny Tummies Delights 75

Chapter 14 Growing Appetites 83

Chapter 15 Toddlers Tasty Tales 93

Foreword

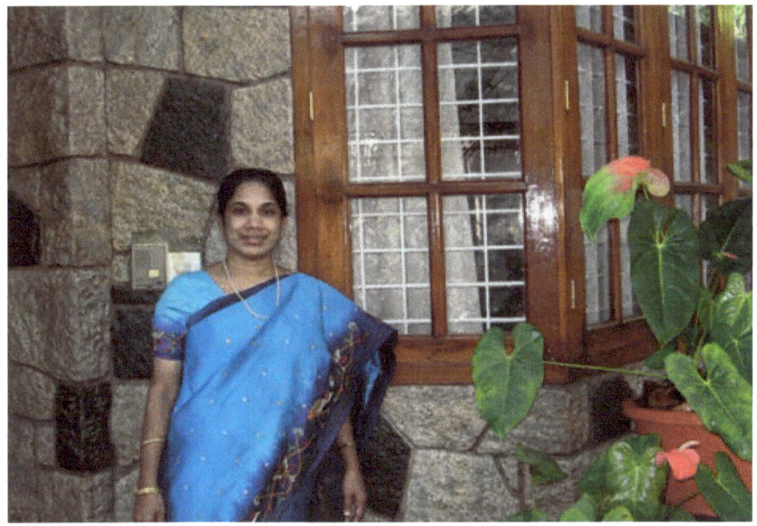

I am extremely delighted to write a foreword for this attractive, handy booklet on 'Nourishing Little Ones: The First Bites: A Comprehensive Guide to Complementary Feeding and Recipe Ideas for 6 Months to 2 Years Children' by Dr. Kalyani Patra, Navi Mumbai. I congratulate her on this succinct compilation in a very lucid manner.

The new slogan is C4 GDP – Complementary Feeding for Growth, Development & Prosperity. Complementary Feeding (CF) is the weakest link in child nutrition. It used to be called 'Weaning', but now this term is abandoned. The term weaning may be used to denote the complete cessation of breastfeeding. CF should be understood as a bridge to be constructed between the phases of liquid to solid diet. In many families, only some thin cereal gruel with added sugar is given to the baby. In some families, different food items are churned in a mixer and given to the child. In India, only around 10% of children aged 6-24 months are getting the 'Minimum Acceptable Diet (MAD)'. Meeting Minimum Dietary Diversity (MDD) and Minimum Meal Frequency (MMF) seems herculean without empowerment. Toddler feeding is yet another big challenge, where eating times become battle times.

The Indian Academy of Pediatrics has urged observing CF Day on the 6th day of the 6th month, June 6th, in order to popularize the timely introduction upon completion of 6 months, capitalizing on the developmental readiness of the baby. It is decided to celebrate the 'Half Birthday and Rice Giving Annaprasan Ceremony' for every baby and start optimum CF. It is important to ensure a well-baby visit at the completion of 6 months in order to empower the family on the 6 attributes of CF: FATVAH. FATVAH represents Frequency, Amount, Texture & Taste, Active Responsive Feeding, and Hygiene. This empowerment is expected to be a boon for the growing babies. Dr. Kalyani has nicely planned the topics in different, well-understandable sections. The booklet includes kitchen-based delicacies, requesting a Social Behavioral Change Communication (SBCC) to look for the right food in the kitchen rather than in the supermarket. The presentation is commendable with respect to content, narration, layout, and so on.

I wish and pray that this book becomes a ready reckoner for many households as well as practicing doctors and dieticians. With all best wishes.

– Dr. Elizabeth KE,
MD, DCH, PhD, FIAP, FRCPCH
Professor & HOD, Pediatrics,
Govt. Medical College, Trivandrum

Preface

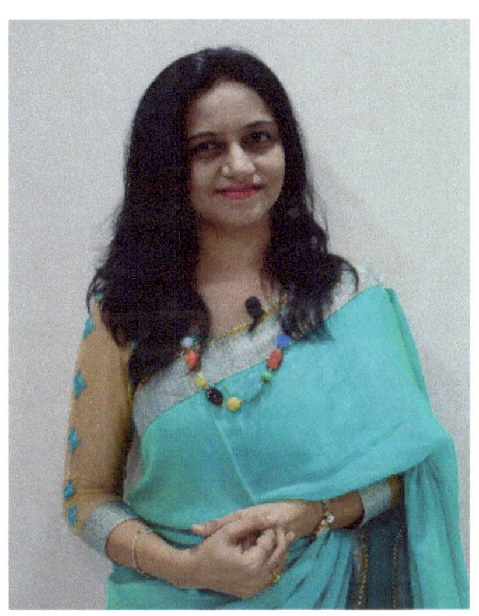

As a pediatrician with several years of experience, I have had the privilege of working closely with countless parents. Through these interactions, it has become evident that there is a significant lack of knowledge and understanding regarding the science of complementary feeding. Many parents, despite their best intentions, hold misconceptions that can inadvertently affect their child's nutrition and health.

One common concern I have observed is the uncertainty about which types of home-cooked foods are appropriate for young children. This gap in knowledge often leads parents to rely on commercially available complementary feeding products, which may not always be the best choice for their child's developing needs.

This book, *Nourishing Little Ones: The First Bites: A comprehensive guide to complementary feeding and Recipe Ideas for 6 months to 2 years children'* is born out of the need to address these gaps. It aims to provide parents with clear, science-based information on complementary feeding, coupled with practical guidance on how to implement this knowledge in their daily lives.

In addition to covering various topics related to complementary feeding, this book also includes a collection of easy-to-prepare recipes. These recipes are designed to help parents offer nutritious, home-cooked meals that can lay a strong foundation for their child's future health.

By equipping parents with the right knowledge and tools, I hope to empower them to make informed decisions about their child's nutrition, fostering healthier eating habits from the very beginning.

– Dr. Kalyani Patra
MBBS, DCH (Gold Medalist), PGDAP
Consultant Pediatrician and Adolescent Expert
Adolescent Care Centre, Kamothe
MGM New Bombay Hospital, Navi Mumbai

Nourishing Little Ones: The First Bites

A Comprehensive Guide to Complementary Feeding and Recipe Ideas

for 6 months to 2 years Children

A handbook for Pediatricians, Parents and Dieticians

DR. KALYANI PATRA

MBBS, DCH (Gold Medalist), PGDAP
Consultant Pediatrician and Adolescent Expert
Adolescent Care Centre and Children's Wellness Clinic, Kamothe
MGM New Bombay Hospital, Navi Mumbai
Executive Board Member, Navi Mumbai IAP (NMAP)
Founder Secretary, Navi Mumbai AHA (NaMAHA)
Centre in charge, Navi Mumbai AACCI, 2024

Dedicated to all Parents, Grand Parents and Care givers

Chapter 1

Introduction

"Little bites today, a healthy life tomorrow."

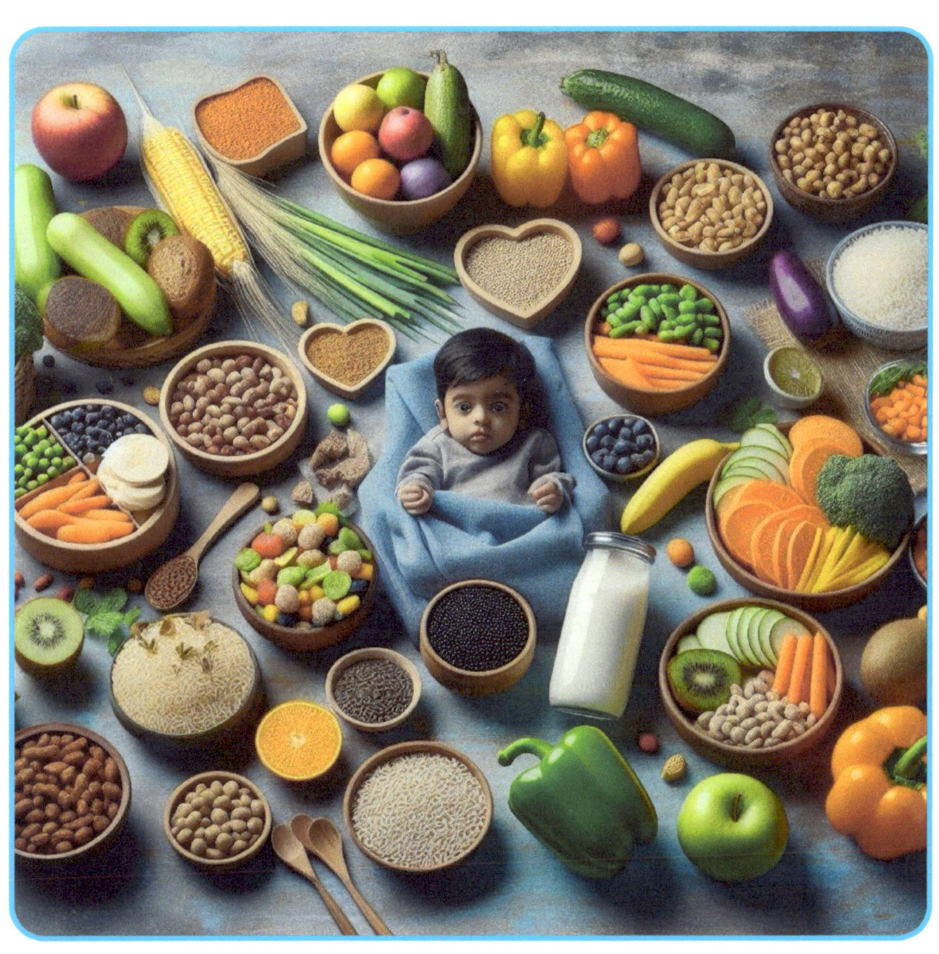

> *"Nourishing our children's bodies and minds is the greatest gift we can give them."*
>
> **– Dr. Christiane Northrup**

Welcome to the world of nourishing your little one through complementary feeding! Introducing solid foods to your infant is a major milestone in their development, marking the transition from exclusive milk feeding to a more diverse diet. This book is your guide to understanding the principles of complementary feeding and providing your baby with the nutrition they need to thrive.

As parents, caregivers, and guardians, we understand the importance of laying a strong nutritional foundation early in life. Complementary feeding, which typically begins around 6 months of age, is a crucial phase that sets the stage for your child's long-term health and eating habits. By introducing a variety of foods at the right time and in the right way, you can support your infant's growth, development, and overall well-being.

In this book, we will explore the fundamentals of complementary feeding, including the timing of introduction, suitable foods, preparation methods, portion sizes, and feeding techniques. You will learn how to ensure that your child receives the essential nutrients for optimal growth and development while also fostering a positive relationship with food.

Whether you are a first-time parent or an experienced caregiver, navigating the world of feeding solids to infants can be both exciting and overwhelming. With the guidance and recipes provided in this book, you will feel empowered to make informed decisions about your child's nutrition and create delicious, balanced meals that your little one will love.

So, grab a spoon and get ready to embark on a culinary adventure as we dive into the wonderful world of complementary feeding for infants. Together, we will explore recipes, tips, and tricks to make mealtime a joyful and nourishing experience for you and your baby.

What is Complementary Feeding?

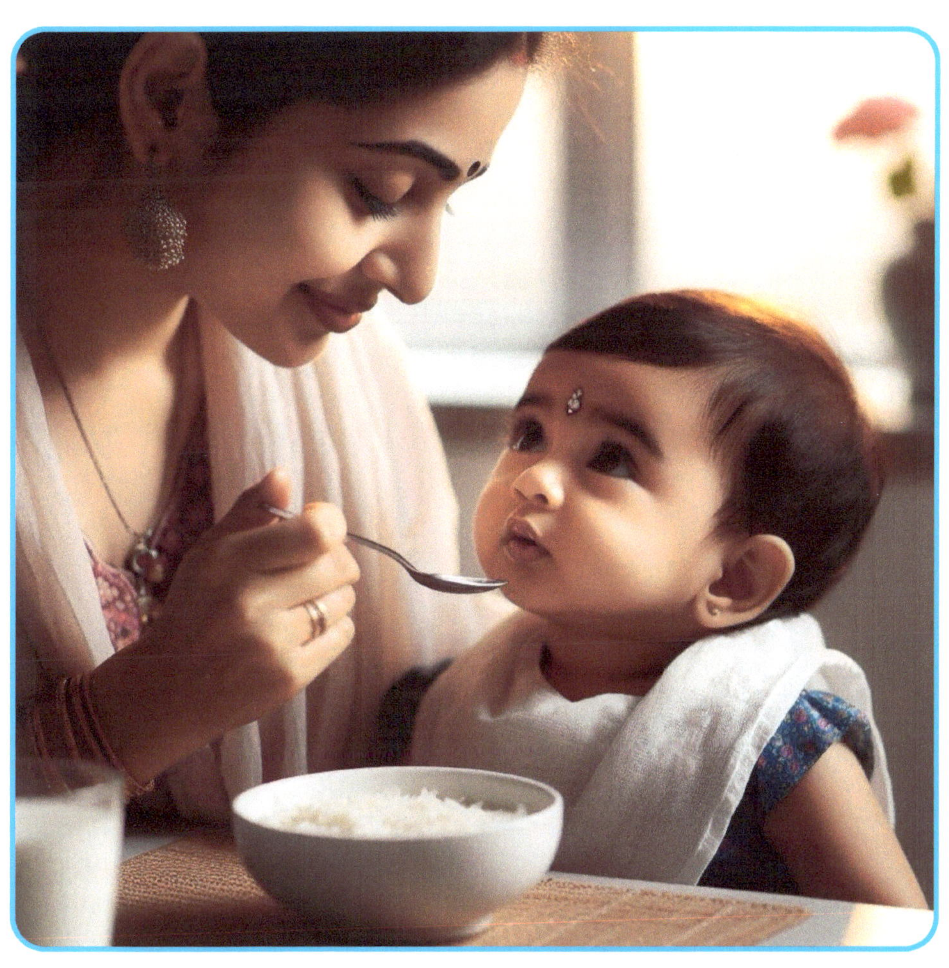

> *"The most important thing we can give our children is a healthy start in life."*
>
> **– Dr. T. Berry Brazelton**

Complementary feeding, previously known as weaning, refers to the introduction of solid foods and liquids other than breast milk into an infant's diet to complement their nutrition. This typically begins around 6 months of age when milk alone may no longer be sufficient to meet all of the infant's nutritional needs. The goal of complementary feeding is to gradually transition the infant from a milk-based diet to a varied diet that includes a range of nutrients essential for their growth and development. Parents or caregivers should introduce a variety of age-appropriate foods while continuing to offer breast milk as an important source of nutrition.

Complementary feeding is a crucial stage in a child's development, bridging the gap between exclusive breastfeeding and family foods.

Key principles for complementary feeding:

1. Duration of Exclusive Breastfeeding and Introduction of Complementary Foods:

    a. Exclusive breastfeeding should continue for the first 6 months of life.

    b. Complementary foods are introduced around 6 months when breast milk alone is no longer sufficient to meet nutritional needs.

2. <u>Continue Breastfeeding:</u>

   a. Continue breastfeeding alongside complementary foods until at least 2 years of age or beyond.

   b. Breast milk remains an essential source of nutrients and immune protection.

3. <u>Practice Responsive Feeding:</u>

   a. Feed infants directly and assist older children.

   b. Feed slowly, patiently, and encourage eating without forcing.

   c. Maintain eye contact and respond to hunger and satiety cues.

4. <u>Attributes of Foods for Complementary Feeding:</u>

   a. Simple and less time-consuming methods to prepare/ cook the foods.

   b. Affordability by the family.

   c. Prefer the regular family food that is locally available and culturally acceptable.

   d. Appealing to the child to encourage them to eat a diverse range of nutritious foods.

5. <u>Safe Preparation and Storage of Complementary Foods:</u>

   a. Ensure hygienic storage and preparation.

   b. Use clean hands and utensils.

   c. Avoid feeding from bottles and teats.

6. <u>Increase the Amount and Nutrient Content of Complementary Foods:</u>

   a. Gradually increase the quantity of complementary foods as the child grows.

   b. Include nutrient-rich foods like fruits, vegetables, grains, and protein sources.

7. <u>Adapt Food Consistency with Age:</u>

   a. Start with soft, mashed foods and progress to thicker textures.

   b. Introduce finger foods as the child develops motor skills (usually by 8 months).

   c. Encourage eating family foods by the end of 1 year.

8. <u>Increase Meal Frequency and Energy Density:</u>

   a. Offer frequent meals (3 main meals and 2-3 snacks) to meet energy needs.

   b. Include energy-dense foods like healthy fats and protein.

9. <u>Nutrient Content of Complementary Foods:</u>

   a. Provide a variety of foods to ensure a balanced intake of vitamins, minerals, and macronutrients.

Remember, complementary feeding is a critical window for establishing healthy eating habits and preventing growth faltering and nutrient deficiencies.

Table describing the Quantity, frequency, and texture of complementary foods

Quantity, frequency, and texture of complementary foods			
Age	**Texture**	**Frequency**	**Average amount of each meal**
6 – 8 months	Begin with mashed foods or thick porridges	Daily 2–3 meals along with frequent breastfeeding	In the beginning, 2–3 tablespoon-full
9 – 11 months	Mashed foods, finely chopped, and foods that can be picked up by baby	Daily 3 meals with continued breastfeeding plus offer 1–2 additional snacks	1/2 cup/bowl (125 mL)
12 months – 2 years	Staple family foods, mashed or chopped (if required)	Daily 3–4 meals with continued breastfeeding plus 1–2 additional snacks	3/4 to one cup/ bowl (250 mL)
Those not being breastfed, give additional 1–2 cups of milk plus 1–2 extra meals daily.			

Source: IAP Parental Guidelines on Complementary Feeding

The Joy of Feeding Your Little One

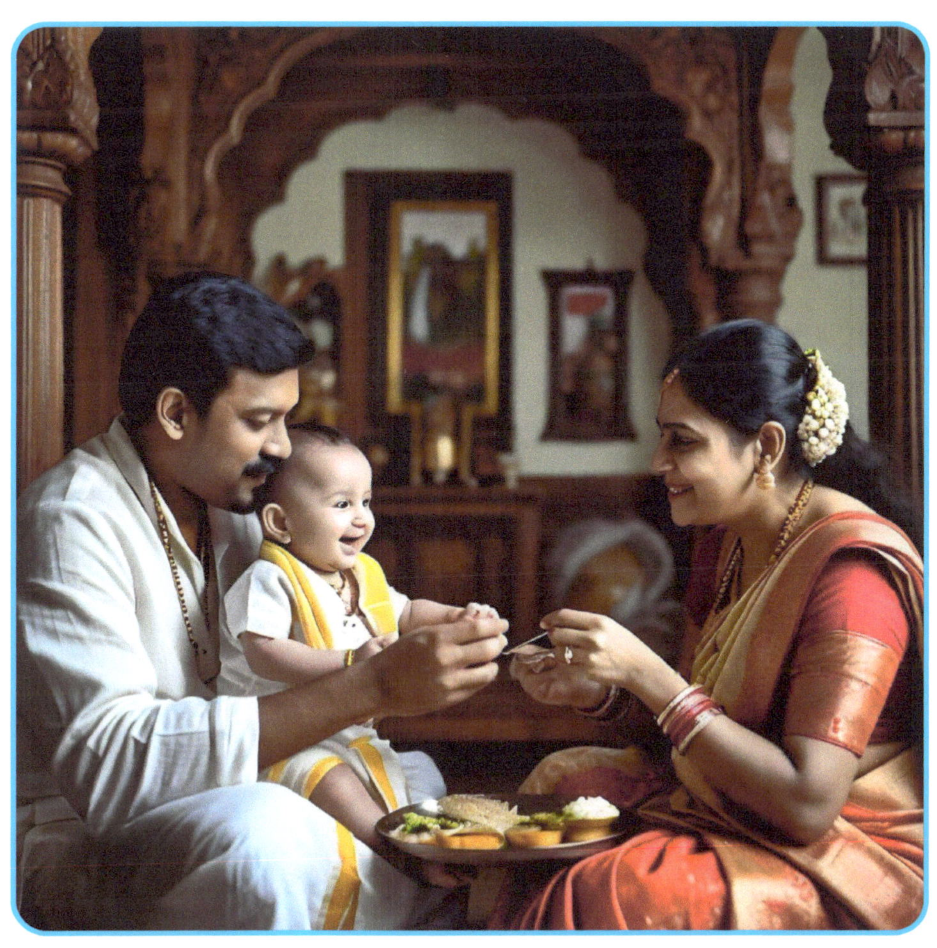

> *"A child's palate is like a canvas, and parents are the artists."*
>
> **– Chef Dan Barber**

<u>Creating a Feeding Environment and Bonding Through Feeding:</u>

Creating a positive feeding environment during this period is vital for fostering healthy eating habits, ensuring adequate nutrition, and supporting emotional and social development.

1. <u>Promotes Healthy Eating Habits:</u>

   a. Establishes Food Preferences: A positive feeding environment encourages children to explore a variety of foods, helping to establish preferences for healthy options early on.

   b. Reduces Picky Eating: Consistent exposure to diverse foods in a stress-free setting can decrease the likelihood of picky eating behaviors.

   c. Encourages Self-regulation: Allowing children to self-feed and decide how much to eat fosters self-regulation and helps prevent overeating.

2. <u>Ensures Adequate Nutrition:</u>

   a. Balanced Diet: A supportive environment ensures that children receive a balanced diet rich in essential nutrients, crucial for growth and development.

   b. Prevents Nutrient Deficiencies: Positive feeding practices reduce the risk of nutrient deficiencies by promoting a varied and nutrient-dense diet.

3. <u>Supports Emotional and Social Development:</u>

   a. Positive Associations with Food: Creating a joyful and relaxed atmosphere around mealtimes helps children develop positive associations with food, which can last a lifetime.

   b. Strengthens Family Bonds: Shared mealtimes provide opportunities for family bonding and communication, enhancing emotional well-being.

   c. Builds Confidence: Encouraging children to try new foods and eat independently builds their confidence and autonomy.

4. <u>Facilitates Developmental Milestones:</u>

   a. Fine Motor Skills: Self-feeding practices, such as picking up small pieces of food, help develop fine motor skills.

   b. Oral Motor Skills: Chewing and swallowing different textures enhance oral motor skills, important for speech development.

5. <u>Reduces Mealtime Stress:</u>

   a. Calm Atmosphere: A calm and patient approach reduces stress for both the child and the caregiver, making mealtimes more enjoyable.

   b. Positive Reinforcement: Encouragement and positive reinforcement can make children feel secure and willing to try new foods.

<u>Strategies for Creating a Positive Feeding Environment:</u>

1. Set a Routine: Establish regular meal and snack times to provide structure and predictability.

2. Create a Pleasant Setting: Ensure a clean, comfortable, and distraction-free eating area.

3. Be Patient and Responsive: Allow children to eat at their own pace and respond to their hunger and fullness cues.

4. Lead by Example: Model healthy eating behaviors and a positive attitude toward food.

5. Involve the Child: Engage children in meal preparation and selection to increase their interest in food.

6. Avoid Pressure: Refrain from pressuring children to eat certain foods or finish everything on their plate.

Creating a positive feeding environment during complementary feeding is foundational for a child's lifelong relationship with food. It promotes healthy eating habits, ensures adequate nutrition, supports emotional and social development, facilitates developmental milestones, and reduces mealtime stress. By adopting strategies that foster a supportive and joyful atmosphere, caregivers can significantly influence their child's growth and well-being, laying the groundwork for a healthy future.

Understanding Your Child's Nutritional Needs

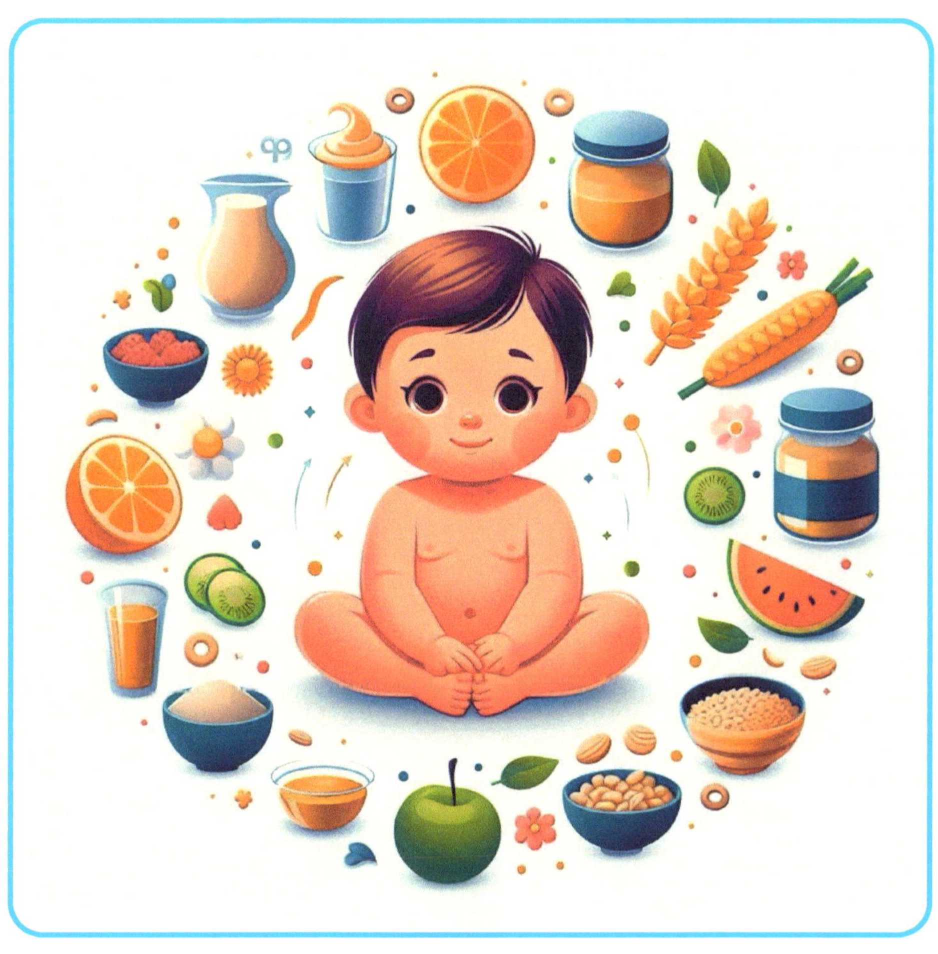

"Teach your children to eat a rainbow, and they'll be eating a rainbow of nutrients."

– Dr. Andrew Weil

Complementary feeding is crucial for meeting the growing nutritional needs of infants, supporting their development, and establishing healthy eating habits. Understanding the role of macronutrients—carbohydrates, proteins, and fats—is fundamental to ensuring a balanced diet.

<u>Essential Nutrients for Infants:</u>

1. Carbohydrates

Importance:

- Primary Energy Source: Carbohydrates are the main source of energy for infants, fueling their rapid growth and high activity levels.
- Brain Development: Glucose, a simple carbohydrate, is essential for brain function and development.
- Digestive Health: Complex carbohydrates provide dietary fiber, which aids in healthy digestion and prevents constipation.

Sources:

- Simple Carbohydrates: Fruits (bananas, apples, pears), vegetables (carrots, sweet potatoes).
- Complex Carbohydrates: Whole grains (rice, millets, and wheat), legumes (lentils, beans), and vegetables (peas, corn).

Guidelines:

- Balanced Intake: Ensure a balance of simple and complex carbohydrates for sustained energy and digestive health.
- Variety: Introduce a variety of carbohydrate sources to expose the child to different tastes and textures.

2. Proteins

Importance:

- Growth and Repair: Proteins are crucial for the growth, repair, and maintenance of tissues, muscles, and organs.
- Immune Function: Proteins help in the production of antibodies and enzymes that support the immune system.
- Development: Amino acids, the building blocks of proteins, are vital for cognitive and physical development.

Sources:

- Animal Proteins: Dairy products, fish, eggs, and meat.
- Plant Proteins: Nuts, lentils, beans, soya, peas, tofu, etc

Guidelines:

- Diverse Sources: Provide a mix of animal and plant proteins to ensure a complete profile of essential amino acids.
- Age-appropriate Portions: Offer small, manageable portions and gradually increase as the child grows.

3. Fats

Importance:

- Energy-Dense: Fats provide a concentrated source of energy essential for infants' rapid growth.

- Brain Development: Essential fatty acids (such as DHA and ARA) are crucial for brain and eye development.
- Absorption of Vitamins: Fats aid in the absorption of fat-soluble vitamins (A, D, E, K).

Sources:

- Healthy Fats: vegetable oil and nut butter
- Animal Fats: Fatty fish (salmon, sardines), full-fat dairy products (yogurt, cheese).
- Plant-based Fats: Flaxseeds, chia seeds, and nuts (for older children or in ground form).

Guidelines:

- Healthy Fats: Focus on providing healthy, unsaturated fats and limit saturated and trans fats.
- Variety of Sources: Include a variety of fat sources to ensure a balanced intake of essential fatty acids.

<u>Essential Micronutrients and Minerals:</u>

1. Iron

- Importance: Iron is crucial for cognitive development and the production of hemoglobin, which carries oxygen in the blood.
- Sources: Green leafy vegetables, jaggery, dates, beetroot, nuts, meat, fish, etc

2. Zinc

- Importance: Zinc supports immune function, cell growth, and repair.
- Sources: Meat, poultry, beans, lentils, chickpeas, and whole grains.

3. Calcium

- Importance: Essential for the development of strong bones and teeth.
- Sources: Dairy products, tofu, fortified plant-based milk, ragi, nuts, and leafy green vegetables.

4. Vitamin D

- Importance: Helps the body absorb calcium and promotes bone health.
- Sources: dairy products, fatty fish (salmon, mackerel), and safe sun exposure. Vitamin D supplements are recommended till 1 year of age (as per your pediatrician's advice).

5. Vitamin A

- Importance: Important for vision, immune function, and skin health.
- Sources: Sweet potatoes, carrots, pumpkin, spinach, and fortified dairy products.

6. Vitamin C

- Importance: Enhances iron absorption, supports the immune system, and acts as an antioxidant.
- Sources: Citrus fruits (oranges, lemons), guava, grapes, amla (Indian gooseberries), strawberries, broccoli, and tomatoes.

Monitoring and Adjusting:

1. Growth and Development

- Regular Check-ups: Schedule regular pediatric check-ups to monitor growth, development, and nutritional status.

- Adjust Diet: Adjust the diet based on the child's growth patterns and any specific nutritional needs identified by the healthcare provider.

2. Parental Guidance

- Educational Resources: Utilize resources from pediatricians, nutritionists, and reputable health organizations to stay informed about best practices in complementary feeding.

Understanding and meeting your child's nutritional needs during complementary feeding is crucial for their growth, development, and long-term health. By offering a variety of nutrient-rich foods, paying attention to textures and portion sizes, and responding to their hunger and fullness cues, parents can ensure a positive feeding experience that lays the foundation for healthy eating habits. Carbohydrates, proteins, and fats each play a vital role in supporting the child's development, making it essential to provide a balanced and varied diet.

Chapter 5

Hygiene Measures

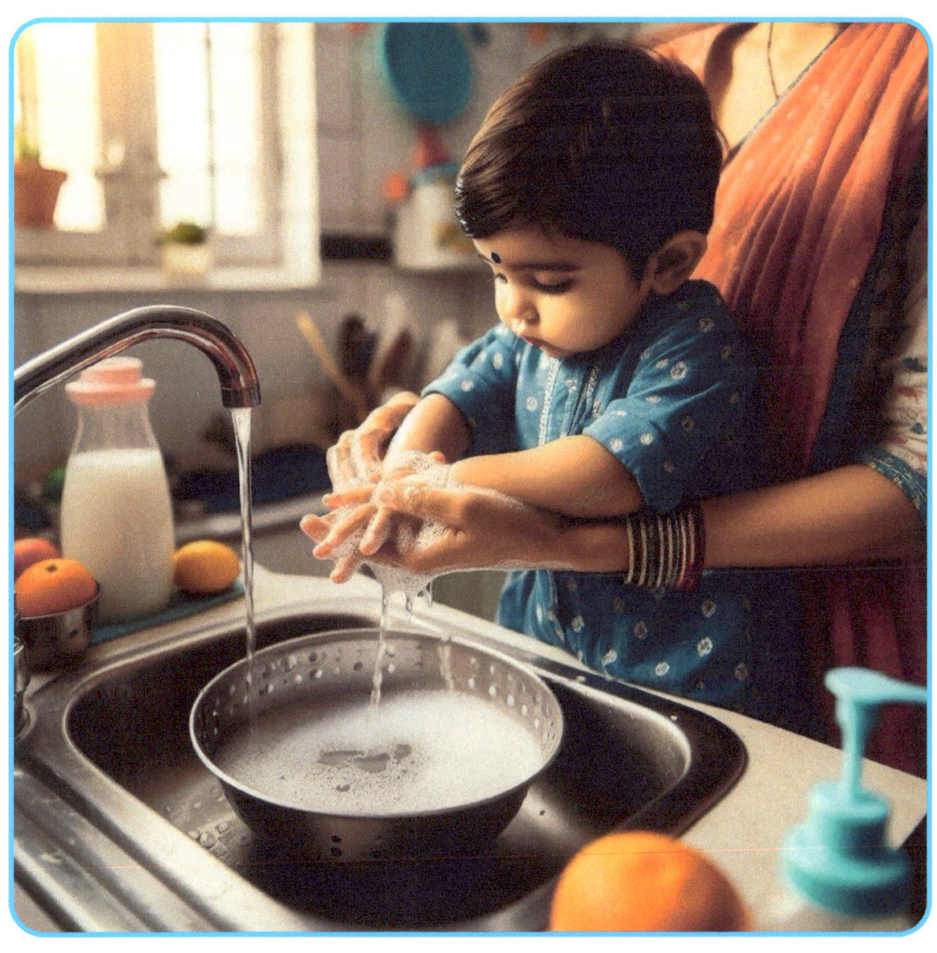

> *"The greatest wealth is health, and the greatest health is cleanliness."*
>
> **– Benjamin Franklin**

In the context of introducing complementary feeding to infants aged 6 months to 2 years, hygiene measures are of paramount importance to ensure the health and well-being of the child. Maintaining a clean and sanitized environment throughout the food preparation and feeding process is crucial in preventing infections and promoting healthy growth and development. This chapter will outline key hygiene measures that caregivers and parents should adhere to when introducing complementary foods to young children.

1. Handwashing:

One of the most critical hygiene practices is handwashing. Caregivers should wash their hands thoroughly with soap and water before preparing food, before feeding the child, and after handling any raw meat, poultry, fish, or eggs. Additionally, make sure to wash the child's hands before meals to prevent the spread of germs.

2. Clean utensils and surfaces:

Ensure that all utensils, such as bowls, spoons, and cups, are clean and sanitized before use. Wash them with hot, soapy water and rinse thoroughly. Avoid using the same utensils as those used for raw meats without proper cleaning. Similarly, clean all food preparation surfaces such as countertops, cutting boards, and high chairs to prevent cross-contamination.

3. Safe food storage:

Properly store complementary foods in airtight containers in the refrigerator to prevent the growth of harmful bacteria. Make sure to label and date containers to keep track of expiration dates. Avoid feeding the child leftovers that have been stored for too long to reduce the risk of foodborne illness.

4. Avoid cross-contamination:

Prevent cross-contamination by keeping raw meats, poultry, and seafood separate from other foods in the refrigerator and during food preparation. Use different cutting boards and utensils for raw and cooked foods to avoid the transfer of bacteria.

5. Safe water supply:

Ensure that the water used for food preparation, cooking, and drinking is safe and free from contaminants. If the safety of the water is questionable, consider boiling water or using filtered water for cooking and preparing infant formula.

6. Proper food handling:

Handle foods with care, especially perishable items such as dairy products, meats, and eggs. Store these foods at the appropriate temperature and never leave them out at room temperature for extended periods. Thoroughly cook meats and eggs to kill any harmful bacteria present.

7. Be cautious with food allergies:

If your child has known food allergies, be extra vigilant about avoiding cross-contact and ensuring that the allergen is not present in any foods being offered as complementary feeding.

8. Maintain a clean feeding environment:

Keep feeding areas clean and free from pests and insects. Regularly clean high chairs, bibs, and any spillages promptly to prevent the growth of bacteria.

By following these hygiene measures diligently, caregivers can help protect their infants as they transition to complementary feeding. Remember, ensuring proper hygiene practices is key to promoting the health and safety of young children during this crucial stage of development.

Recommendations on Sugar and Salt

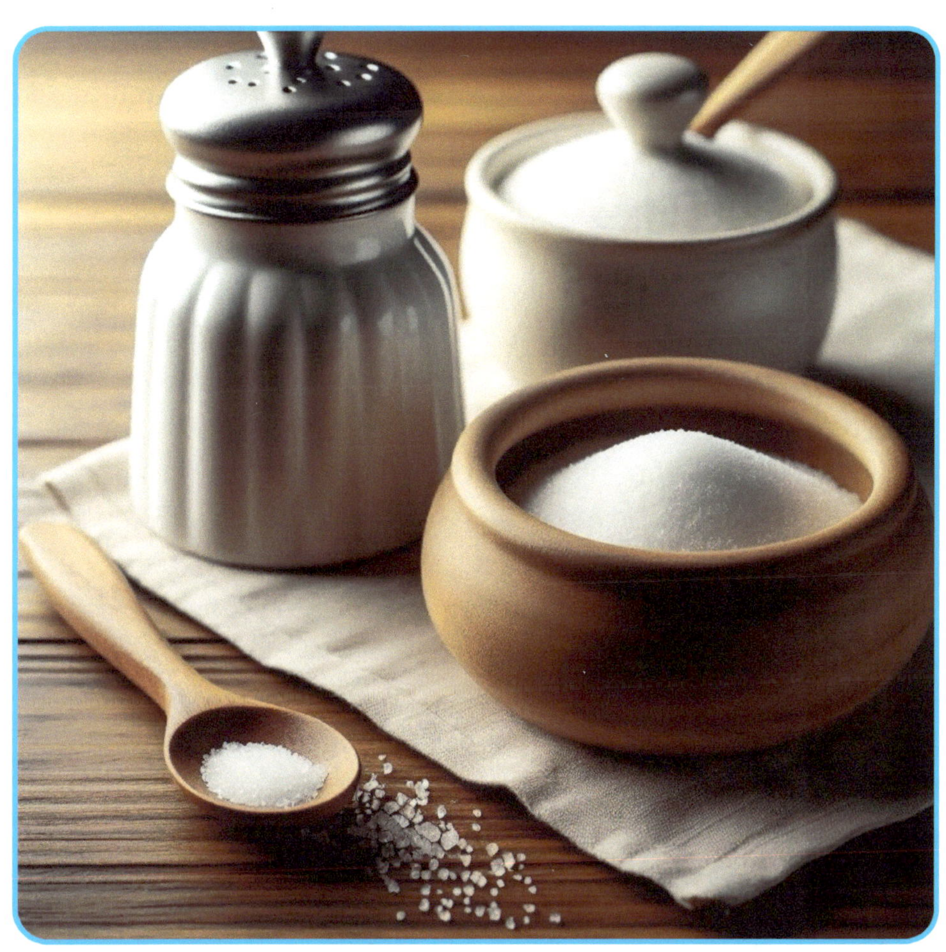

> *"Sugar and salt are the 2 most addictive substances in the world, and we're addicted to both of them."*
>
> **– Dr. Andrew Weil**

As parents, one of the most common dilemmas we face during the complementary feeding journey is how much sugar and salt to introduce into our children's diets. While sugar and salt may enhance the taste of foods, it is crucial to approach these additives mindfully to ensure the optimal health and development of our little ones. In this chapter, we will delve into recommendations regarding sugar and salt consumption for children aged 6 months to 2 years.

<u>Sugar Intake Recommendations:</u>

1. Limit Added Sugar:

The Indian Academy of Pediatrics (IAP) and the World Health Organization (WHO) recommend restricting the intake of added sugars for children below 2 years of age. Added sugars refer to the sugars added during food processing or preparation, such as sweetened beverages, cakes, and candies. Excessive consumption of added sugars is linked to various health issues like obesity, dental problems, and a preference for sweet foods.

2. Natural Sugars:

Instead of added sugars, opt for foods containing natural sugars like fruits. Fruits not only provide natural sweetness but also offer essential nutrients like vitamins, fiber, and antioxidants necessary for a child's growth.

3. Avoid Honey:

It is important to avoid giving honey to infants under the age of one year due to the risk of infant botulism, a rare but serious illness caused by bacteria found in honey.

Salt Intake Recommendations:

1. Monitor Sodium Intake:

Salt, which is a major source of sodium, is essential for the body in small quantities. However, excessive salt consumption in childhood can lead to health concerns like high blood pressure and kidney problems later in life. It is crucial to monitor and limit the intake of salt in your child's diet.

2. Avoid Processed Foods:

Processed and packaged foods often contain high amounts of hidden salt. It is advisable to prepare fresh meals at home using natural ingredients to have better control over the salt content in your child's diet.

3. Flavoring Alternatives:

Instead of salt, consider using herbs, spices, and natural flavorings to enhance the taste of your child's meals.

Practical Tips for Parents:

1. Read Labels:

When purchasing packaged foods, carefully read the labels to identify hidden sugars and salts. Choose products with lower sugar and salt content or opt for homemade alternatives.

2. Lead by Example:

Children often mimic their parents' eating habits. As caregivers, it is essential to model healthy eating behaviors by consuming balanced meals low in sugar and salt.

3. Consult Healthcare Providers:

If you have concerns about your child's sugar and salt intake, do not hesitate to seek guidance from your child's pediatrician or a registered dietitian. They can provide tailored recommendations based on your child's individual needs.

In conclusion, being mindful of sugar and salt consumption is crucial for promoting a healthy diet and overall well-being in children aged 6 months to 2 years. By prioritizing whole, nutrient-dense foods and limiting added sugars and salt, parents can pave the way for healthy eating habits that will benefit their children in the long run.

The Correct Use and Importance of Oil and Ghee

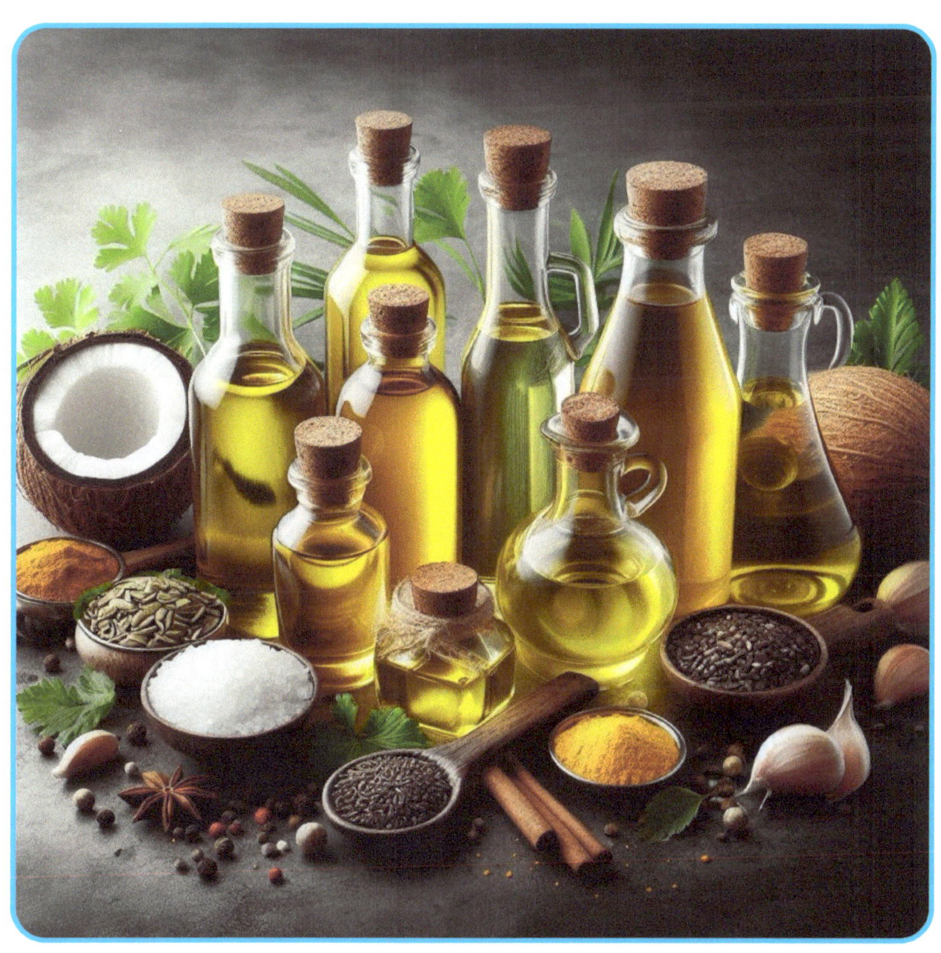

"Ghee kindles agni (digestive fire), nourishes the body, and promotes mental clarity."

– Charaka Samhita

In India, oils and ghee (clarified butter) hold a significant place in traditional diets and culinary practices. They are not only important for enhancing the taste and texture of foods but also serve as crucial sources of energy and essential fatty acids. Understanding the correct use and benefits of oils and ghee in complementary feeding is vital for ensuring the nutritional adequacy and health of Indian children.

Importance of Fats in Complementary Feeding:

Fats are a critical component of an infant's diet, especially during the complementary feeding phase. They provide a concentrated source of energy, support brain development, and aid in the absorption of fat-soluble vitamins (A, D, E, and K). Given the rapid growth and development that occurs in the first 2 years of life, incorporating healthy fats like oils and ghee into a child's diet is essential.

<u>Types of Oils and Ghee:</u>

1. Oils:

- Vegetable Oils: These include oils derived from seeds, nuts, and fruits. Common vegetable oils used in Indian households include mustard oil, sesame oil, coconut oil, and groundnut (peanut) oil.
- Refined Oils: These are processed oils like sunflower oil, soybean oil, and rice bran oil, which are commonly used for cooking.

2. Ghee:

- Traditional Ghee: Made by simmering butter and removing the milk solids, traditional ghee is rich in saturated fats and has a distinct flavor.
- Cultured Ghee: Made from cultured butter (butter that has been fermented), it is believed to have additional probiotic benefits.

<u>Benefits of Oils and Ghee in Complementary Feeding:</u>

1. Energy Source:

- High-Caloric Density: Both oils and ghee are energy-dense foods, providing more calories per gram compared to carbohydrates and proteins. This is particularly important for infants and young children who have high energy needs but small stomach capacities.

2. Essential Fatty Acids:

- Omega-3 and Omega-6: Oils like mustard oil, flaxseed oil, and walnut oil are rich in essential fatty acids, particularly omega-3 and omega-6, which are crucial for brain development and overall growth.
- Medium-Chain Triglycerides (MCTs): Coconut oil contains MCTs, which are easily digestible and quickly converted into energy, making them ideal for young children.

3. Vitamin Absorption:

- Fat-Soluble Vitamins: The presence of fats in the diet aids in the absorption of fat-soluble vitamins such as A, D, E, and K. Ghee, in particular, is a good source of vitamin A and E.

4. Gut Health:

- Probiotic Benefits: Cultured ghee can support gut health by introducing beneficial bacteria.
- Anti-Inflammatory Properties: Both ghee and certain oils (like olive oil) have anti-inflammatory properties that can promote overall health and well-being.

5. Flavor and Palatability:

- Taste Enhancement: The addition of ghee and oils can enhance the flavor and palatability of foods, encouraging better acceptance of a variety of foods among children.

Correct Use of Oils and Ghee:

1. Age-Appropriate Introduction:

- Starting at Six Months: Small amounts of oils and ghee can be introduced when the child begins complementary feeding, typically around 6 months of age.
- Gradual Increase: Start with small quantities (about half a teaspoon) and gradually increase as the child grows and their diet diversifies.

2. Balanced Intake:

- Moderation: While oils and ghee are beneficial, they should be used in moderation to avoid excessive calorie intake and ensure a balanced diet.
- Variety: Use a variety of oils to provide a range of fatty acids and nutrients. For instance, alternate between mustard oil, sesame oil, and coconut oil.

3. Cooking Methods:

– Low-Heat Cooking: Use oils and ghee for low to medium-heat cooking to preserve their nutritional qualities. High-heat cooking can destroy beneficial fatty acids and create harmful compounds.

– Raw Use: Some oils, like peanut oil and olive oil, can be used raw (e.g., drizzled over salads or mixed into purees) to maximize their health benefits.

4. Food Preparation:

– Incorporating into Foods: Add ghee or oil to mashed vegetables, dals (lentils), khichdi (a mixture of rice and lentils), and porridges to increase the energy density of these foods.

– Consistency and Texture: Ensure that the added fats do not make the food too greasy or difficult to swallow. The consistency should be appropriate for the child's developmental stage.

Cultural and Traditional Perspectives:

1. Ayurveda:

– Ghee in Ayurveda: Ghee is highly regarded in Ayurvedic medicine for its nourishing and healing properties. It is believed to improve digestion, boost immunity, and support brain function.

– Traditional Practices: Incorporating small amounts of ghee in a child's diet aligns with traditional practices that have been followed for generations.

2. Regional Variations:

- Cultural Preferences: Different regions in India have unique preferences for specific oils and ghee, influenced by local cuisine and availability.
- Embracing these practices can make complementary feeding culturally relevant and acceptable.

Addressing Common Concerns:

1. Saturated Fats:

- Balanced Diet: While ghee is high in saturated fats, it can be part of a balanced diet when consumed in moderation. Focus on a variety of fat sources, including unsaturated fats from oils.
- Quality Over Quantity: Choose high-quality ghee made from grass-fed cows, and avoid overconsumption to maintain a healthy balance.

2. Allergies:

- Monitoring: Introduce new oils and ghee gradually and monitor for any allergic reactions. While rare, some children may have sensitivities to certain types of oils.
- Consultation: If there are concerns about allergies or intolerances, consult a pediatrician before introducing new fats into the diet.

Oils and ghee are important components of complementary feeding, providing essential nutrients, energy, and aiding in the absorption of fat-soluble vitamins. Their correct use enhances the nutritional quality of a child's diet, supports growth and development, and aligns with cultural and traditional practices in India. By incorporating these fats in moderation and variety, parents and caregivers can ensure a balanced and nutritious diet for their children, laying the foundation for lifelong health and well-being.

Chapter 8

Spice Recommendations

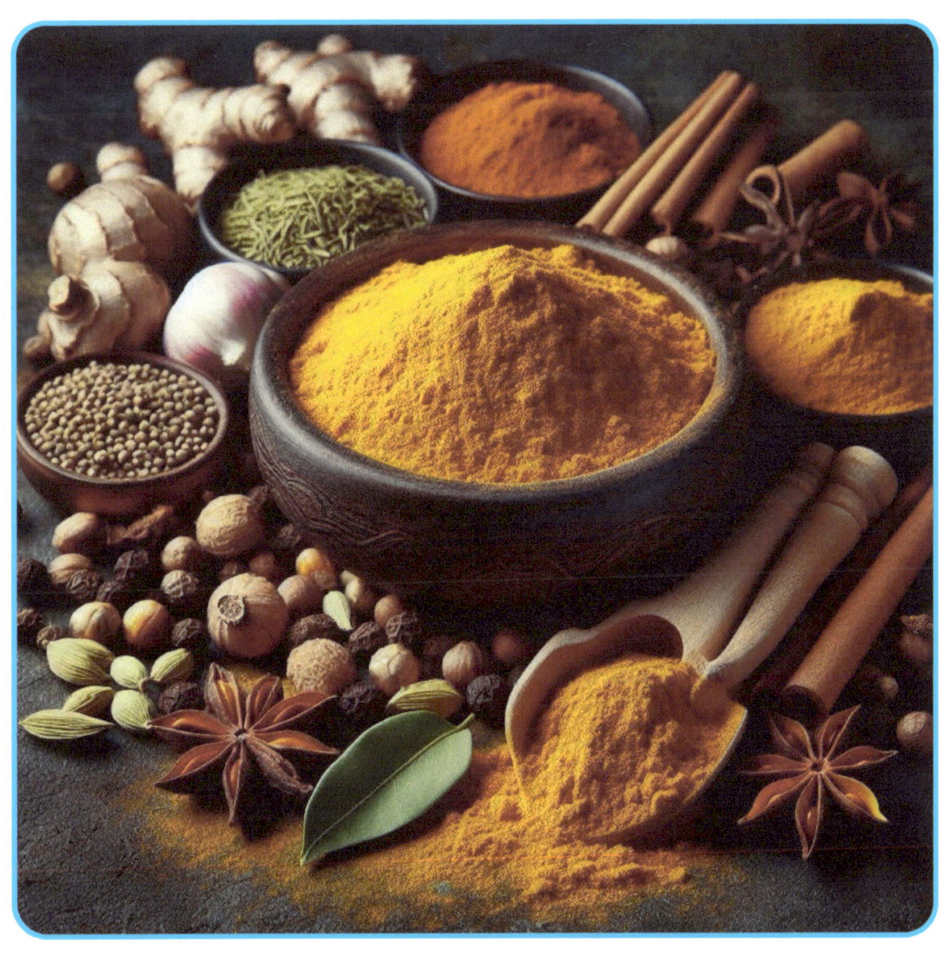

> *"Spices are the magic ingredients that transform food into medicine."*
>
> **– Dr. Vasant Lad**

Spices play a central role in Indian cuisine, not only for their flavor-enhancing properties but also for their potential health benefits. When introducing complementary foods to infants in India, incorporating spices thoughtfully can enhance palatability, aid digestion, and introduce infants to the rich cultural heritage of Indian culinary traditions. This chapter explores the safe and beneficial use of spices in complementary feeding.

<u>Importance of Spices in Complementary Feeding:</u>

1. Flavor Enhancement

   – Palatability: Spices add variety and depth of flavor to foods, making them more appealing to infants who are transitioning from milk to solid foods.
   – Cultural Heritage: Introducing infants to spices familiarizes them with traditional Indian flavors and cultural practices from an early age.

2. Digestive Benefits

   – Promoting Digestion: Certain spices have digestive properties that can help alleviate common gastrointestinal issues such as gas and bloating.
   – Anti-inflammatory Effects: Spices like turmeric and ginger have anti-inflammatory properties that may support overall gut health.

3. Nutritional Value

- Antioxidants: Many spices are rich in antioxidants, which help protect cells from damage and support immune function.
- Vitamins and Minerals: Spices can contribute small amounts of essential vitamins and minerals to an infant's diet.

Safe and Recommended Spices for Infants:

1. Cumin (Jeera)

- Benefits: Cumin aids digestion, reduces flatulence, and has a mild, earthy flavor.
- Usage: Add a pinch of roasted and ground cumin to khichdi, dals, and vegetable purees.

2. Turmeric (Haldi)

- Benefits: Turmeric is known for its anti-inflammatory properties and contains curcumin, which has antioxidant benefits.
- Usage: A tiny pinch can be added to savory dishes like rice and lentil porridge (khichdi) or vegetable stews.

3. Coriander (Dhania)

- Benefits: Coriander seeds aid digestion and have a mild, citrusy flavor that is gentle for infants.
- Usage: Use ground coriander in vegetable purees, soups, and lentil soups (dal).

4. Fennel (Saunf)

- Benefits: Fennel seeds help relieve colic and digestive discomfort in infants.

- Usage: Infuse water with crushed fennel seeds or add a small amount to soups and rice dishes.

5. Cardamom (Elaichi)

- Benefits: Cardamom aids digestion and adds a sweet, aromatic flavor to foods.
- Usage: Use a tiny amount of ground cardamom in fruit purees, rice pudding (kheer), and yogurt.

6. Ginger (Adrak)

- Benefits: Ginger aids digestion and can help alleviate nausea.
- Usage: Use a small amount of grated or ground ginger in soups, vegetable dishes, and teas (for older infants).

7. Asafoetida (Hing)

- Benefits: Asafoetida aids digestion and is often used to reduce gas and bloating.
- Usage: A tiny pinch of powdered asafoetida can be added to lentil soups (dal) or vegetable dishes.

8. Cinnamon

- Benefits: Cinnamon not only adds flavor but is also rich in antioxidants and has anti-inflammatory properties.
- Usage: It can be added to a variety of dishes such as oatmeal, yogurt, or even pureed fruits.

Guidelines for Introducing Spices:

1. Start Gradually

- Timing: Introduce spices gradually once the infant has accepted basic foods like rice cereal, pureed fruits, and vegetables.

- Quantity: Start with a very small amount (a pinch or less) and gradually increase as the child becomes accustomed to new flavors.

2. Monitor Reactions

- Allergies: Watch for any signs of allergies or sensitivities when introducing new spices.
- Digestive Issues: Monitor how the infant responds to spices known for their digestive properties, adjusting quantities as needed.

3. Preparation Methods

- Roasting and Grinding: Roasting and grinding spices enhances their flavor and makes them easier to digest.
- Infusions: Infuse water or milk with spices like fennel or cardamom for added flavor and potential health benefits.

Cultural and Practical Considerations:

1. Traditional Practices

- Family Recipes: Incorporate family recipes and traditional methods of spice usage to maintain cultural heritage.
- Regional Variations: Embrace regional variations in spice usage to expose infants to diverse flavors and culinary traditions.

2. Health and Safety

- Quality: Use high-quality spices that are fresh and free from contaminants.
- Consultation: If there are concerns about allergies or health conditions, consult a pediatrician before introducing new spices.

Introducing spices in complementary feeding can enhance flavor and aid digestion. By following safe guidelines, starting gradually, and monitoring reactions, parents can incorporate spices effectively into their child's diet, supporting both health and cultural heritage from an early age. Spices not only add culinary richness but also contribute to the nutritional value of meals, making them an integral part of a balanced and varied diet for growing infants.

Chapter 9

Guide for Water Intake

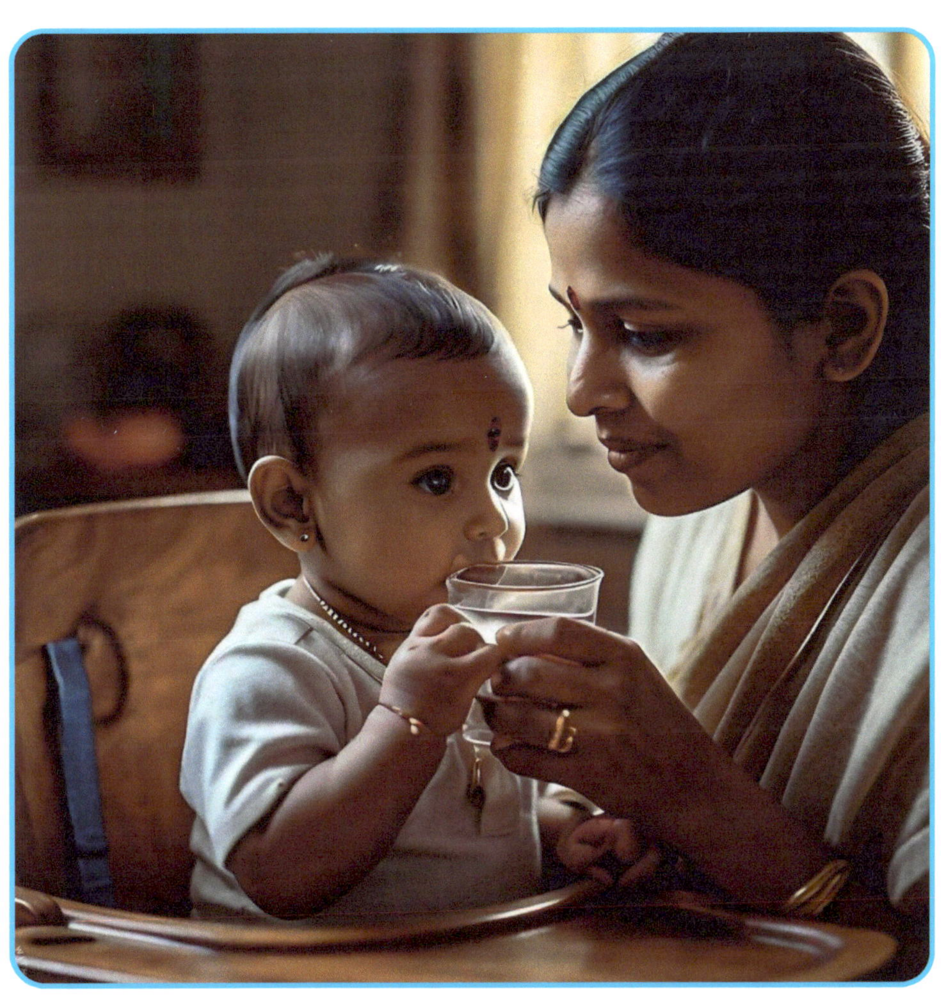

"Water is the driving force of all nature."

– Leonardo da Vinci

Water is an essential nutrient for children, and its importance cannot be overstated during complementary feeding. As infants transition from exclusive breastfeeding to solid foods, water plays a critical role in maintaining proper hydration and supporting overall growth and development. In this chapter, we will discuss the importance of water in complementary feeding, how to offer water to children aged 6 months to 2 years, and tips for encouraging water intake.

Importance of Water:

- Maintains fluid balance and hydration
- Supports digestion, nutrient absorption, and is essential for overall growth and development
- Helps regulate body temperature
- Promotes healthy urinary tract function

Offering Water:

- Start offering water at 6 months alongside solid foods
- Use a clean, sterile cup or bottle
- Offer water after feeding solid foods to help with swallowing and digestion
- Gradually increase water intake as the child grows

Tips for Encouraging Water Intake:

- Make water easily accessible and offer it frequently throughout the day
- Mix water with breast milk to create a familiar taste

- Make it fun by using colorful cups or straws
- Set a good example by drinking water yourself

Water is a vital component of complementary feeding, and its importance should not be overlooked. By understanding the significance of water and following the guidelines and tips outlined in this chapter, caregivers can help ensure their children stay properly hydrated and support their overall growth and development.

Chapter 10

Common Challenges and Solutions

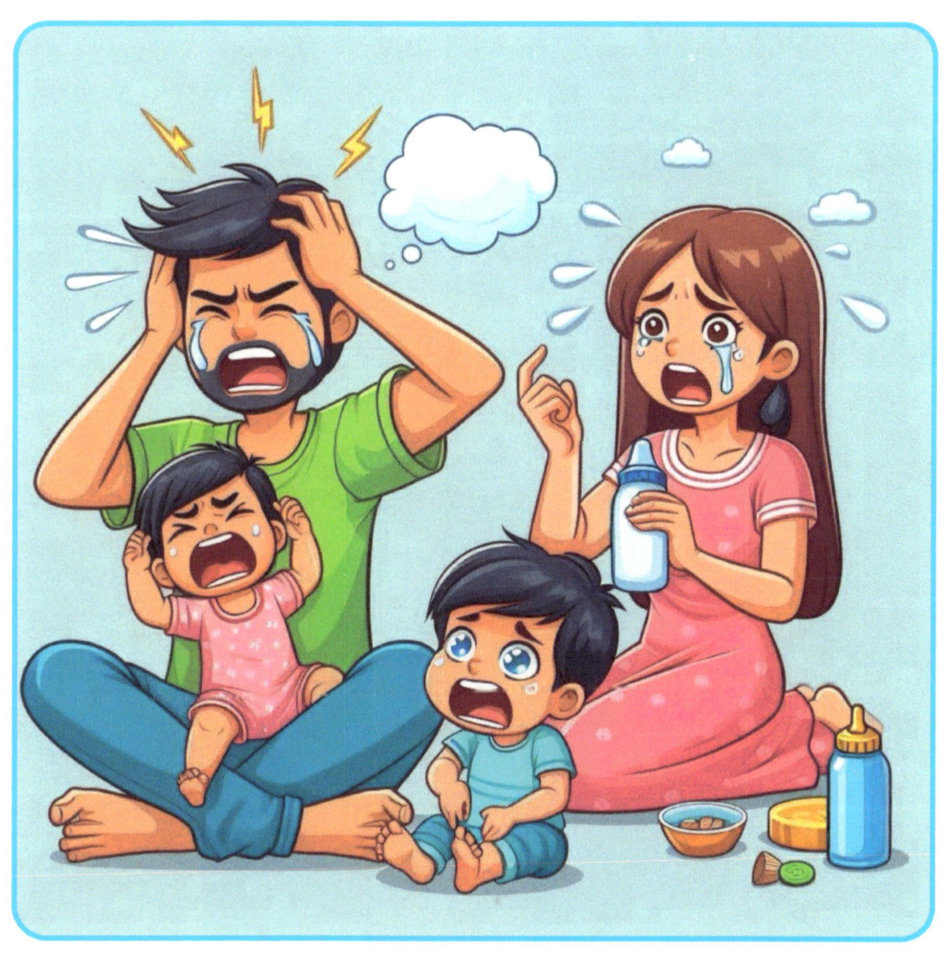

> *"The habits we form from childhood often stick with us for life."*
>
> **– Dr. William Sears**

Parents and caregivers often encounter several challenges. Addressing these challenges effectively can ensure a smooth transition and promote healthy eating habits.

1. Refusal to Eat New Foods

Challenges:

- Fear of New Foods (Food Neophobia): Many children are naturally cautious about new foods and may refuse to try them.
- Texture Sensitivity: Some children may be sensitive to the textures of new foods, leading to refusal.

Solutions:

- Repeated Exposure: Offer new foods multiple times without pressure. It may take several exposures before a child accepts a new food.
- Variety of Textures: Introduce a range of textures gradually, starting with smooth purees and progressing to lumpier foods.
- Positive Reinforcement: Praise the child for trying new foods, even if they don't eat much. Avoid negative reactions or forcing them to eat.

2. Picky Eating

Challenges:

- Limited Diet: Children may prefer a small selection of foods and refuse to eat others, leading to a nutritionally imbalanced diet.
- Routine Resistance: Changes in routine or unfamiliar environments can exacerbate picky eating behaviors.

Solutions:

- Offer Choices: Provide a few healthy options at each meal to give the child some control over what they eat.
- Consistent Mealtime Routine: Maintain a regular meal and snack schedule to establish predictable eating times.
- Modeling Behavior: Eat a variety of foods in front of the child to encourage them to try different foods.

3. Inadequate Nutrient Intake

Challenges:

- Nutrient Deficiencies: Limited food acceptance can lead to deficiencies in essential nutrients such as iron, zinc, and vitamins.
- Balanced Diet: Ensuring a balanced diet with all necessary nutrients can be challenging.

Solutions:

- Nutrient-Dense Foods: Offer foods rich in essential nutrients, such as leafy greens, lean proteins, and fortified cereals.
- Supplements: Consult a pediatrician about appropriate supplements if necessary.

- Mixing Foods: Incorporate nutrient-rich ingredients into familiar foods (e.g., adding pureed vegetables to pasta sauce).

4. Choking Hazards

Challenges:

- Small Objects: Young children are at risk of choking on small, hard, or round foods.
- Inadequate Chewing Skills: Children may not chew food thoroughly, increasing the risk of choking.

Solutions:

- Appropriate Food Preparation: Cut food into small, manageable pieces and avoid foods known to be choking hazards (e.g., whole grapes, nuts).
- Supervision: Always supervise children while they eat and encourage them to eat slowly and chew thoroughly.
- Texture Progression: Gradually introduce lumpier textures to help children develop their chewing skills.

5. Parental Anxiety and Stress

Challenges:

- High Expectations: Parents may feel stressed if their child doesn't eat as expected or if they worry about nutritional adequacy.
- Feeding Battles: Mealtimes can become battlegrounds if there's pressure for the child to eat certain foods.

Solutions:

- Stay Calm: Maintain a relaxed attitude toward feeding to create a positive environment.

- Realistic Expectations: Understand that it's normal for children to have fluctuating appetites and preferences.
- Professional Support: Seek advice from pediatricians or nutritionists to alleviate concerns and receive tailored guidance.

6. Allergies and Intolerances

Challenges:

- Food Allergies: Introducing new foods carries the risk of allergic reactions.
- Food Intolerances: Some children may have intolerances that cause digestive discomfort.

Solutions:

- Detailed discussion in the next chapter

Navigating the challenges of complementary feeding requires patience, persistence, and a positive approach. By addressing common issues such as food refusal, picky eating, and nutritional concerns with effective strategies, parents and caregivers can foster a healthy, enjoyable feeding experience. Ensuring a supportive and flexible environment during this critical period is essential for the child's growth, development, and long-term relationship with food.

Understanding Food Allergies

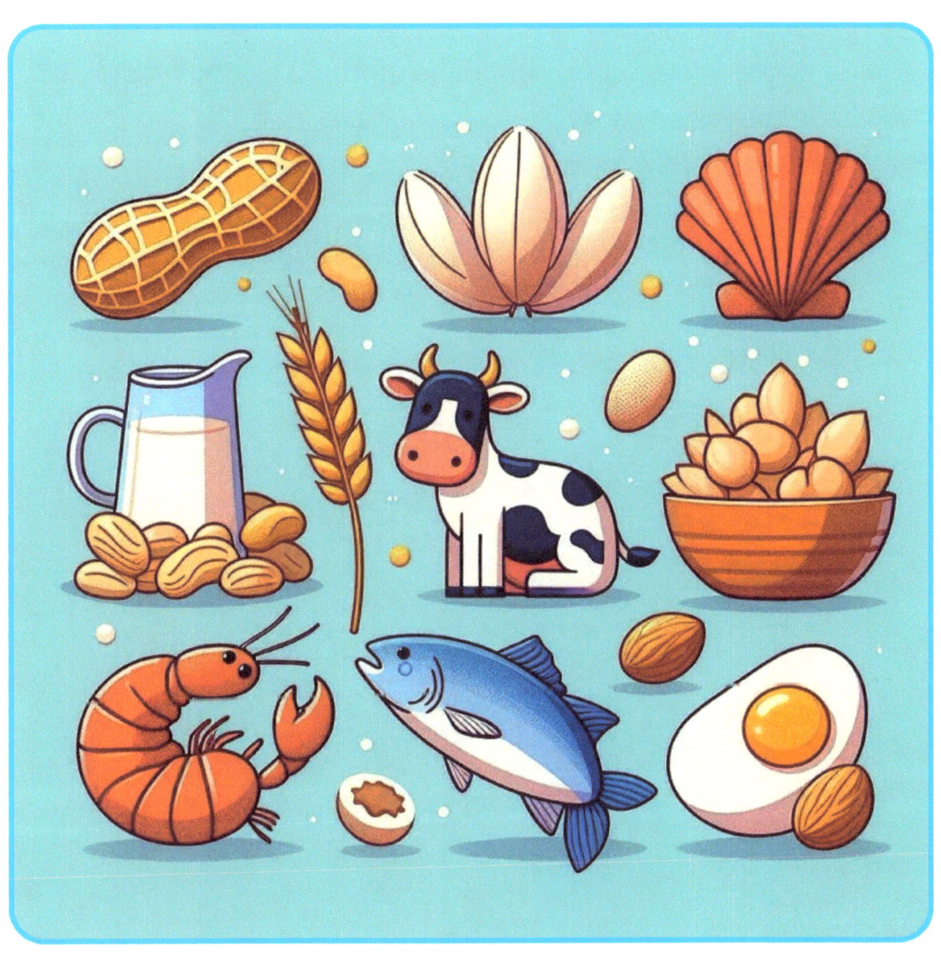

> *"Knowledge is power, and when it comes to food allergies, knowledge can be lifesaving."*
>
> **– Dr. Michael Pistiner**

Food allergies are a growing concern among parents, particularly when introducing complementary foods to infants. This chapter aims to provide parents with comprehensive information on understanding, identifying, and managing food allergies during complementary feeding.

What are Food Allergies?

- Food allergies occur when the immune system mistakenly identifies certain proteins in foods as harmful and triggers an allergic reaction.
- These reactions can range from mild to severe and can affect the skin, digestive system, respiratory system, and cardiovascular system.

Common Food Allergens:

1. Milk

2. Eggs

3. Peanuts

4. Tree Nuts

5. Soy

6. Wheat

7. Fish

8. Shellfish

<u>Identifying Food Allergies:</u>

1. Symptoms to Watch For

    – Skin Reactions: Hives, eczema, swelling of the lips, face, and eyes.
    – Digestive Issues: Vomiting, diarrhea, abdominal pain, and sometimes constipation.
    – Respiratory Symptoms: Wheezing, stridor (noisy inhalation), coughing, shortness of breath.
    – Severe Reactions: Anaphylaxis, which is a medical emergency characterized by a combination of the following symptoms: extensive hives, difficulty breathing, a drop in blood pressure, and loss of consciousness.

2. Timing of Symptoms

    – Immediate Reactions: Symptoms usually appear within minutes to a few hours after eating the allergen.
    – Delayed Reactions: Some reactions may take several hours to develop, particularly with gastrointestinal symptoms.

3. Allergy Testing

    – Consult a pediatrician: If you suspect your child has a food allergy, consult a pediatrician who may recommend allergy testing or a pediatric allergist referral.

<u>Managing Food Allergies:</u>

1. Introduction of Allergenic Foods

    – Early Introduction: Introduce common allergenic foods gradually and one at a time while monitoring for reactions.

- Allergenic Foods Timing: Start introducing them after the child has successfully tolerated basic foods like cereals, fruits, and vegetables.

2. Reading Labels

  – Ingredients: Carefully read food labels to avoid hidden allergens, especially in processed foods.
  – Cross-Contamination: Be aware of potential cross-contamination in foods that are processed in facilities handling allergens.

3. Home-Cooked Meals

  – Control Ingredients: Preparing meals at home allows better control over ingredients and reduces the risk of exposure to allergens.
  – Substitutions: Use allergen-free substitutes in case of allergy to a particular food (e.g., almond milk instead of animal milk) in recipes.

4. Breastfeeding Considerations

  – Maternal Diet: If breastfeeding, the mother's diet can affect the infant, though rarely (e.g., animal milk and egg).
  – Avoid allergenic food consumption in the mother's diet if the child shows reactions to breast milk.

<u>Emergency Plan:</u>

  – Recognize Symptoms: Educate yourself and caregivers on how to recognize and respond to allergic reactions.
  – Adrenaline/Epinephrine Injection: For severe allergies, keep an adrenaline/epinephrine injection ready on hand

and know how to use it. (Get information from your pediatrician)

<u>Cultural and Dietary Considerations:</u>

Traditional Indian Foods

- Legumes and Pulses: Common in Indian diets, they can be allergenic. Introduce them cautiously.
- Spices: While not common allergens, spices like mustard can cause reactions in some children.

<u>Myths and Misconceptions:</u>

1. Delayed Introduction

   - Myth: Delaying the introduction of allergens can prevent allergies.
   - Fact: Early introduction (around 6 months) of allergenic foods may help reduce the risk of developing food allergies.

2. Outgrowing Allergies

   - Myth: Children always outgrow food allergies.
   - Fact: Some children outgrow allergies, while others do not. Regular monitoring and consultation with a healthcare provider are essential.

3. Allergen-Free Diets

   - Myth: Completely avoiding allergens will cure food allergies.
   - Fact: There is no cure for food allergies. Management involves avoiding known allergens and being prepared for accidental exposure.

Understanding and managing food allergies during complementary feeding is crucial for ensuring the health and safety of children. By recognizing common allergens, identifying symptoms, and implementing effective management strategies, parents can navigate this challenging aspect of feeding with confidence. Embracing traditional Indian foods and cultural practices, while staying informed about modern nutritional guidelines, can help create a balanced and allergen-aware diet for growing infants.

Unhealthy Diet and Beverages

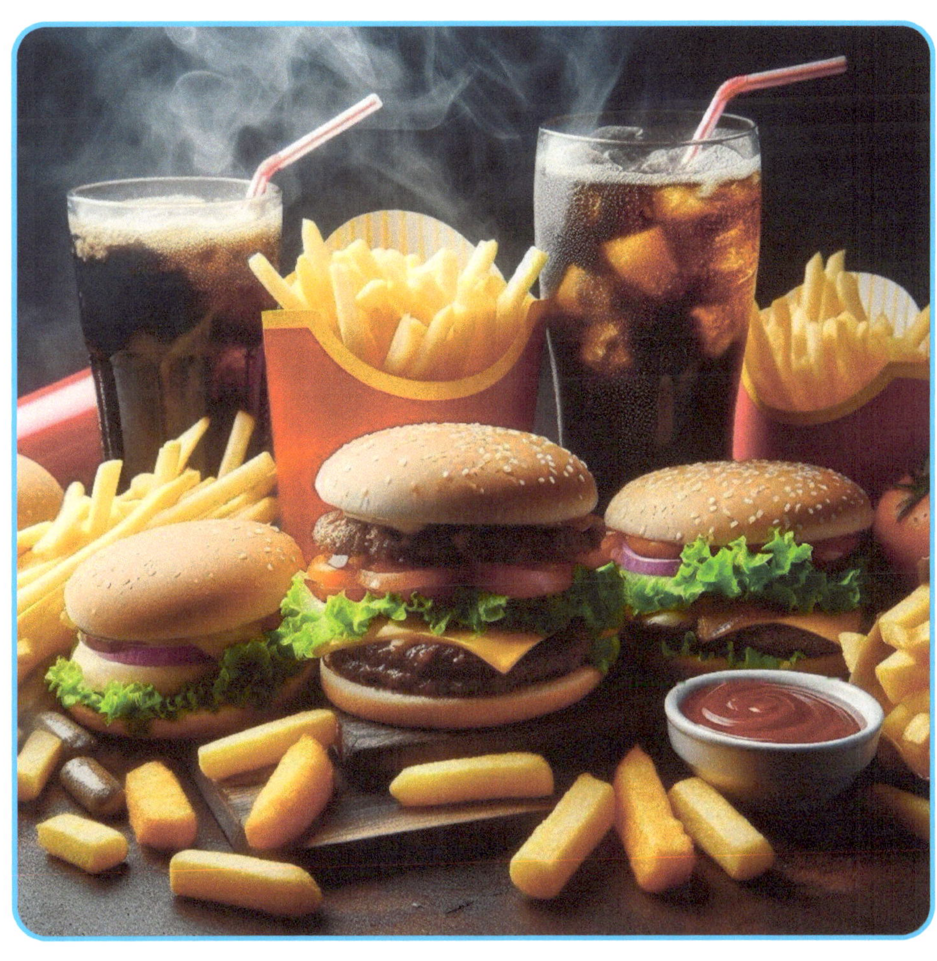

"Healthy eating isn't about deprivation, it's about nourishment."

– Jill Blakeway

In the formative years between 6 months and 2 years, a child's diet plays a pivotal role in their growth, development, and lifelong health. While complementary feeding introduces a variety of nutritious foods, it is equally important to recognize and avoid unhealthy dietary practices that can hinder natural development. This chapter delves into the detrimental effects of unhealthy foods and beverages and offers guidance on making healthier choices for young children.

The Impact of Unhealthy Diets

Unhealthy foods and beverages can significantly affect a child's physical and cognitive development. These effects range from obesity and dental problems to impaired brain function and poorer immune responses. Overconsumption of unhealthy foods at a young age can also set the stage for lifelong unhealthy eating habits.

<u>Common Unhealthy Foods and Beverages:</u>

1. Sugary Foods and Drinks:

   – Sugary Snacks and Desserts: Candies, cookies, cakes, and pastries are often high in sugar and low in nutrients. Regular consumption can lead to tooth decay, obesity, and the development of a preference for sweet foods.

   – Sugary Beverages: Sodas, fruit-flavored drinks, and sweetened juices are loaded with sugars and offer little to no nutritional benefit. They can displace more nutritious beverages like breast milk or water and contribute to excessive caloric intake.

2. High-Sodium Foods:

- Processed Foods: Chips, canned soups, and instant noodles often contain high levels of sodium. Excessive sodium intake can affect kidney function and lead to high blood pressure later in life.
- Fast Foods: These foods are often high in sodium, unhealthy fats, and calories while being low in essential nutrients.

3. Unhealthy Fats:

- Trans Fats and Saturated Fats: Foods like fries and certain baked goods contain unhealthy fats that can lead to cardiovascular disease even from a young age.

4. Low-Nutrient Foods:

- Processed Meats: High in sodium and often lack the required nutrients for a growing child.
- Snack Foods: Offer empty calories and can replace more nutrient-dense options such as fruits, vegetables, and whole grains.

Beyond Physical Health: Cognitive and Behavioral Impact:

Research indicates that diets high in sugar and unhealthy fats can impair cognitive development. The excessive consumption of these foods can lead to problems with memory, attention, and learning capacity. Behavioral issues such as hyperactivity have also been linked to high sugar intake.

<u>Strategies to Avoid Unhealthy Foods and Beverages:</u>

1. Reading Labels:

    –   Always check the nutritional labels on foods and beverages. Avoid products with high amounts of added sugars, sodium, and unhealthy fats.

2. Home-Cooked Meals:

    –   Preparing meals at home allows full control over the ingredients, ensuring that children receive balanced and nutritious meals.

3. Healthy Alternatives:

    –   Substitute unhealthy snacks with fresh fruits, vegetables, and whole grain options. Offer water or diluted pure fruit juices instead of sugary drinks.

4. Limiting Fast Food:

    –   Minimize trips to fast food restaurants and consider healthier options when dining out.

5. Setting a Positive Example:

    –   Children often mimic adult behavior. Consuming healthy foods and beverages yourself will encourage your child to follow suit.

Education and Awareness

Educating caregivers about the potential harm of unhealthy diets is crucial. Public health campaigns and community programs can provide valuable information and resources to families to guide them in making better nutritional choices.

Tiny Tummies Delights

nutrient - packed recipes for

infants 6 months to 8 months of age

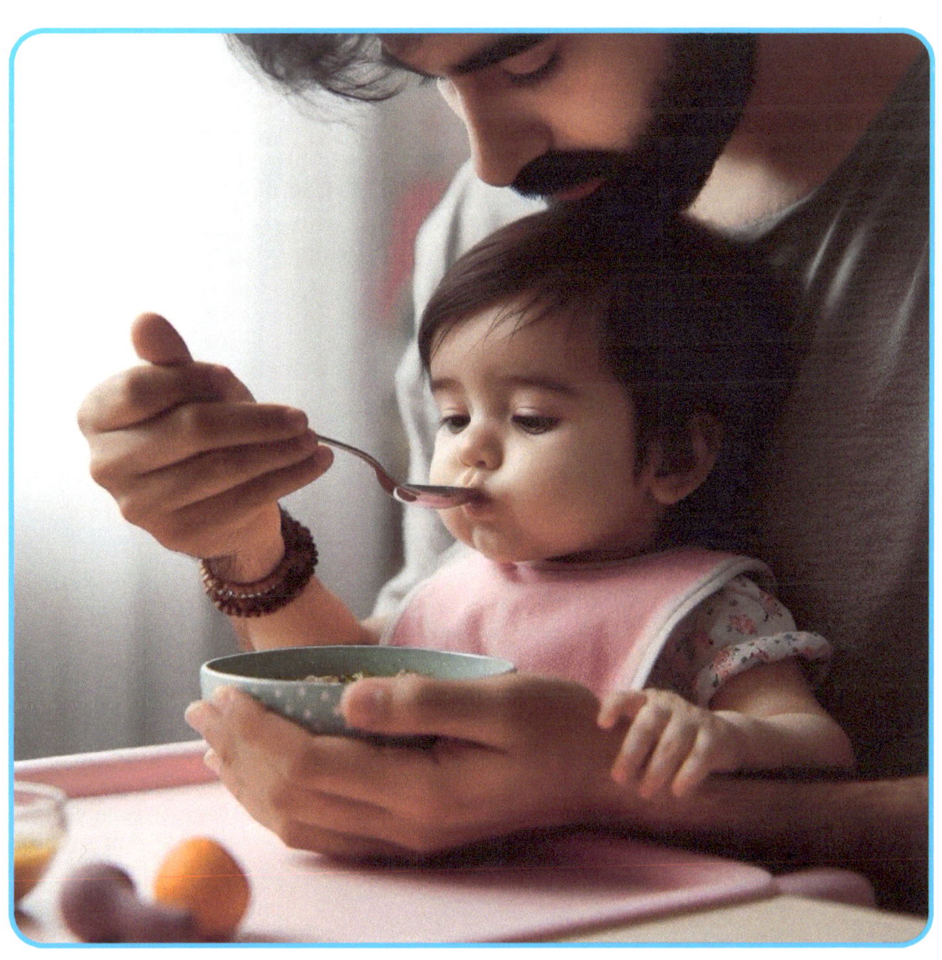

> *"The most important thing we can give our children is a healthy start in life."*
>
> **– Dr. T. Berry Brazelton**

At 6-8 months, your baby is ready to start exploring new tastes and textures. This period marks the beginning of complementary feeding, alongside continued breastfeeding. Here's how to identify your baby's readiness and support their development.

Signs of Readiness:

1. Sitting Up with Support: Your baby can sit upright with minimal support.

2. Good Head Control: Your baby can hold their head steady.

3. Interest in Food: Your baby shows curiosity about what you're eating, reaching out for food.

4. Mouth Movements: Your baby can move food from the front to the back of their mouth to swallow.

Benefits:

1. Nutritional Needs: Complementary foods provide essential nutrients like iron and zinc, which are not sufficiently supplied by breast milk or formula alone after 6 months.

2. Developmental Milestones: Introducing different textures helps develop oral motor skills necessary for chewing and speaking.

3. Taste Exploration: Early exposure to a variety of flavors can help develop a more diverse palate.

Feeding Tips:

1. Start Slow: Introduce one new food at a time, waiting 3-5 days before adding another to monitor for allergies.

2. Smooth Purees: Begin with smooth, single-ingredient purees, gradually increasing texture as your baby gets used to eating.

3. Small Quantities: Offer small amounts of food on a soft spoon, allowing your baby to explore the taste and texture.

4. Be Patient: Allow your baby to eat at their own pace without forcing them. It's normal for them to play with the food and make a mess.

Starting complementary feeding between 6-8 months is a critical step in your baby's development. It provides essential nutrients, supports developmental milestones, and introduces your baby to a variety of tastes and textures. Follow your baby's cues, be patient, and make mealtimes enjoyable. With your support, your baby will thrive on this new adventure of taste and nutrition.

Remember, every child is unique, so adapt these guidelines to your baby's individual needs and pace. Enjoy this exciting journey of exploring new tastes and textures together!

Here are a few complementary feeding recipes for between the ages of 6 to 8 months:

APPLE PUREE:

- Peel and core an apple.
- Cut it into chunks and cook it with a little water until it's soft.
- Blend it into a smooth puree.

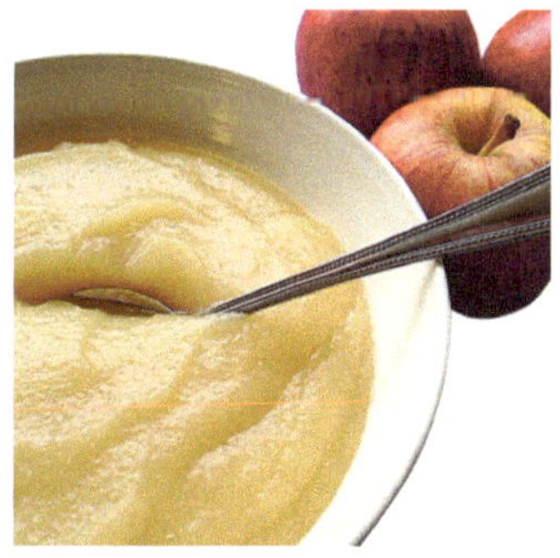

MASHED BANANA:

- Choose a ripe banana.
- Peel it and mash it with a fork until it's smooth.

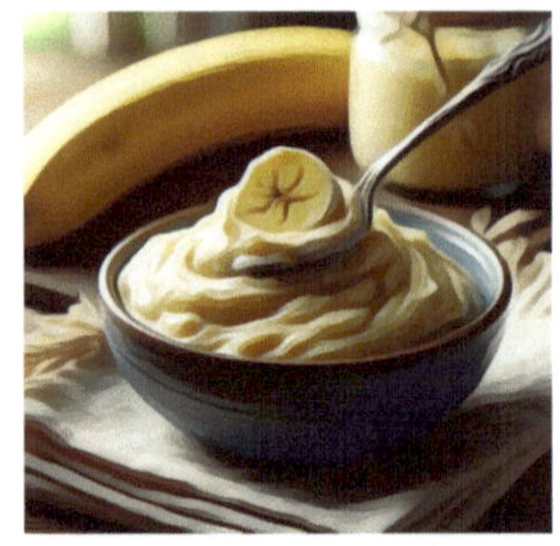

SWEET POTATO MASH:

Ingredients:

- 1 medium sweet potato
- Water for boiling
- A small amount of butter or ghee (optional)
- A pinch of cardamom powder (optional)

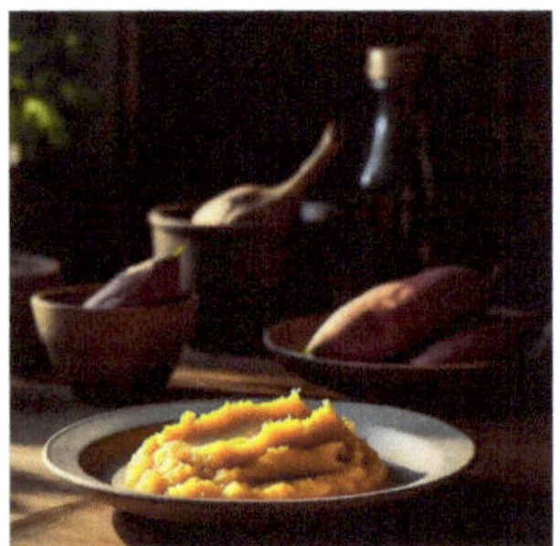

Instructions:

- Peel and chop the sweet potato into small chunks.
- Cover the chunks with water in a saucepan and boil until tender, which should take about 15 minutes.
- Drain the water and add a small amount of butter or ghee if desired, for added flavor and healthy fats.
- Mash using a masher or hand blender until smooth.
- If using, sprinkle a pinch of cardamom powder for flavor and mix well.
- Once fully cooled, you can serve this to your baby. Sweet potatoes are rich in beta-carotene, vitamins, and fiber, making them an excellent food for babies. You can adjust the consistency by adding water or breastmilk.

RICE CEREAL:

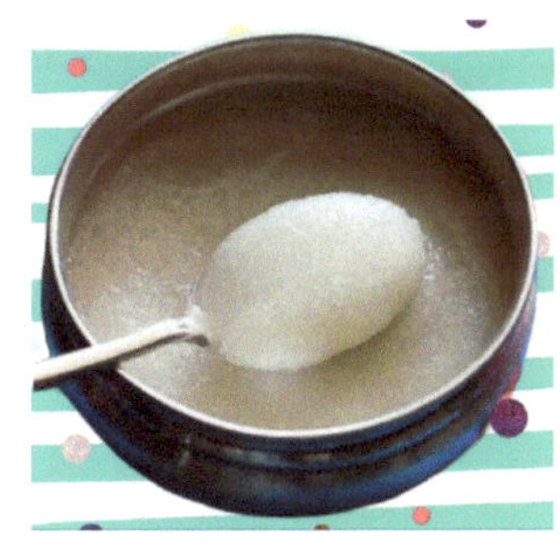

- Wash and dry roast a small amount of rice until it's aromatic.
- Grind it into a fine powder.
- Cook one tablespoon of this powder with water until it's cooked and has a porridge-like consistency.

CARROT PUREE:

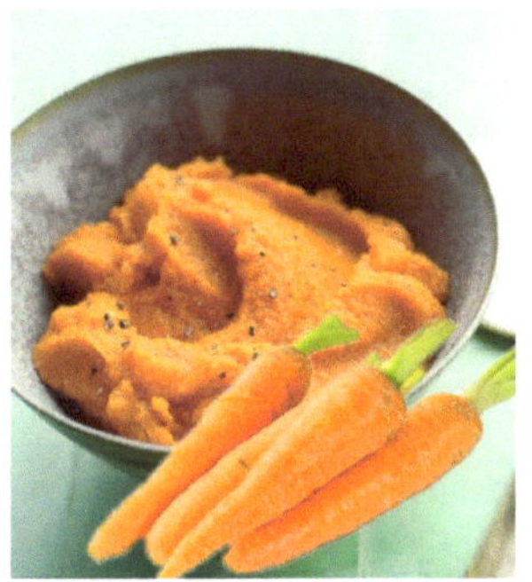

- Peel and chop carrots into small pieces.
- Steam or boil until tender.
- Blend into a smooth puree and add water if necessary.

RAGI HALWA:

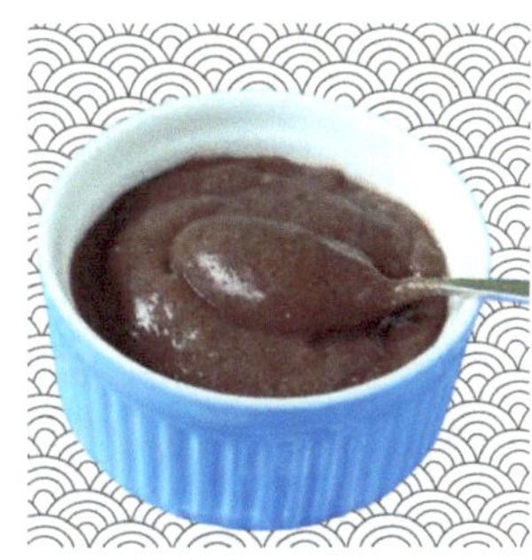

- Dissolve 2 tablespoons of ragi powder in 1 cup of water to make a lump-free batter.
- Cook on low to medium flame, stirring continuously for 2-3 minutes.
- Add the banana puree and ghee, mix well, and cook for another 1-2 minutes until you reach the desired consistency.

HOMEMADE RICE MOONG DAL CEREAL POWDER:

Making homemade cereal powder using rice and moong dal is a great way to provide nutritious options for your little one. Here's a simple recipe for Rice Moong Dal Cereal Powder:

Rice Moong Dal Cereal Powder Recipe:

Ingredients:

- 1/2 cup parboiled (preferable)/ routine white rice
- 1/4 cup moong dal (split green gram)
- 1/8 teaspoon cumin seeds

Instructions:

- Wash the rice and moong dal thoroughly.
- Dry them under the sun or in the shade for about 1 hour until they're completely dry.
- In a pan, dry roast the dried rice, moong dal, and cumin seeds over low flame until the rice is hot to touch and slightly puffy, and the moong dal turns golden here and there.
- Switch off the flame and let it cool.
- Grind the roasted rice, moong dal, and cumin seeds into a fine powder using a mixer.
- Allow the powder to cool completely and store it in an airtight container.

This homemade rice moong dal cereal powder can be used to make instant khichdi for your baby.

MOONG DAL KHICHDI:

Ingredients:

- 2 tbsp rice moong dal cereal powder
- 1 cup water
- A pinch of cumin seeds (optional)
- A tiny pinch of pepper (if the baby is above 8 months old)

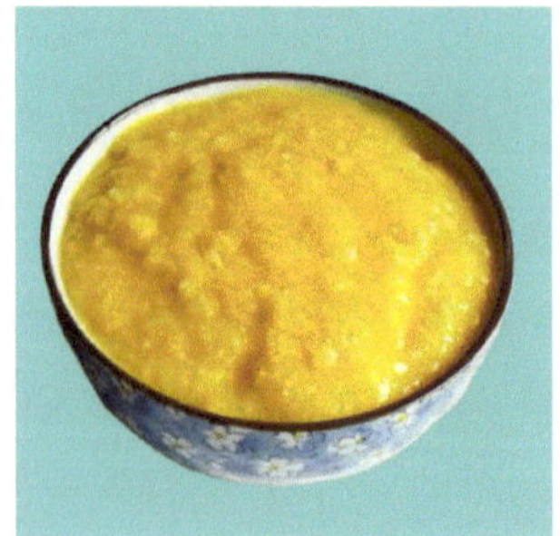

Instructions:

- Mix the cereal powder with water to avoid lumps.
- Cook on low flame until it reaches a saucy consistency.
- Let it cool slightly and feed while it's warm to your baby.

Quick fix:

- You can also add chopped vegetables like carrot, pumpkin, green peas or bottle guard Pressure cook for 2-3 whistles; it reduces the cooking time. Also add ghee before serving to make it complete healthy meal for your baby.

<u>FRUITS:</u>

You can also introduce the following fruits to your baby:

- Apple and Pear: Gentle on the stomach and can be given as a puree or steamed.
- Chikoo: Well ripe chikoo are high in fibers; good for gut.
- Papaya: Ripe papaya is soft and easy to digest.
- Pomegranate: Can be given as juice; rich in iron and other micronutrients.
- Muskmelon: Soft and juicy, ideal for hydration.
- Avocado: Full of healthy fats, perfect for baby's growth.
- Peaches: Can be steamed and pureed.

Always ensure the fruits are ripe and mash or puree them to the right consistency for your baby. It's also important to introduce one fruit at a time and wait for 3 days to check for any allergic reactions.

"The earlier they start, the healthier they'll be."

Growing Appetites

wholesome meals for 9-11 months

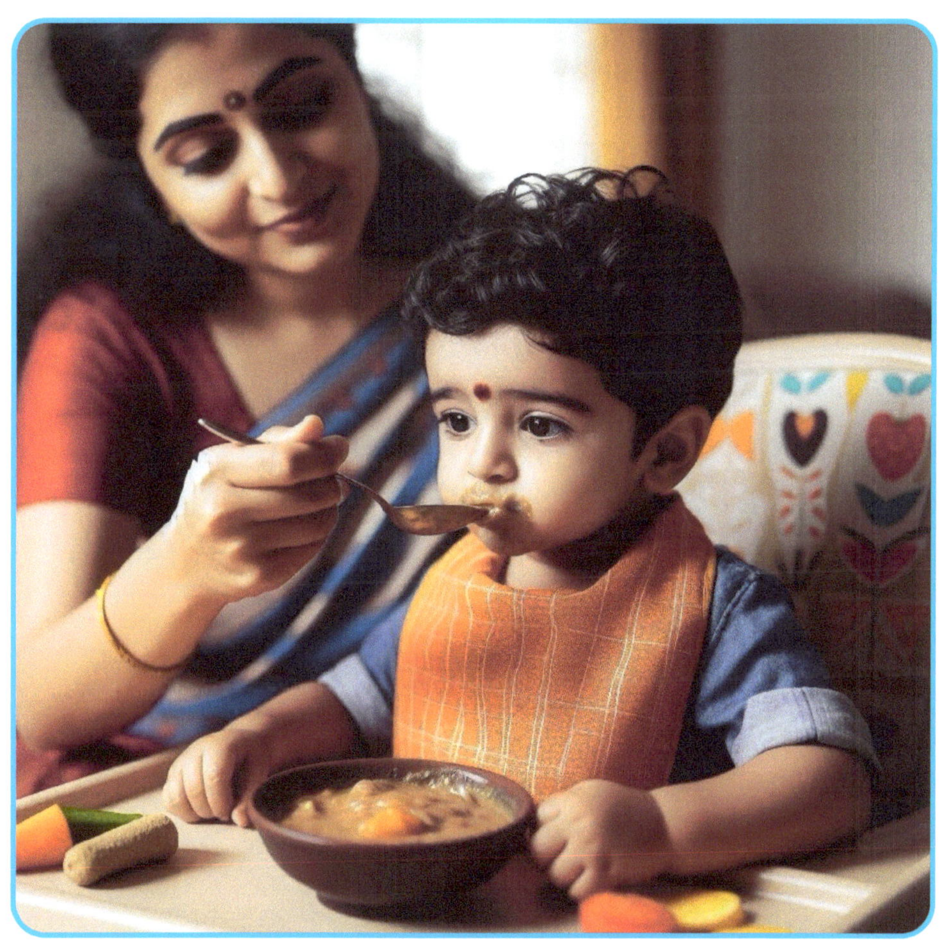

*"Healthy eating is a habit that can be developed
and enjoyed at any age."*

– Dr. Jane Travis

By 9-11 months, your baby has made significant progress in their developmental milestones. Here's what to expect and how to support their readiness for more complex complementary feeding:

Signs of Readiness:

1. Improved Hand-Eye Coordination: Your baby can now pick up small pieces of food using their thumb and forefinger (pincer grasp).

2. Chewing Ability: Enhanced ability to chew and manage a variety of textures.

3. Increased Independence: Your baby may show a desire to self-feed with fingers or a spoon.

Benefits:

1. Fine Motor Skills: Encouraging self-feeding helps develop fine motor skills.

2. Oral Development: Chewing different textures aids in oral development, preparing for speech.

3. Exploration and Learning: Handling and tasting new foods supports sensory exploration and cognitive development.

Feeding Tips:

1. Variety and Texture: Offer a range of foods with different textures, such as soft fruits, cooked vegetables, small pieces of meat, and finger foods.

2. Encourage Self-Feeding: Allow your baby to use their hands and a spoon, even if it gets messy.

3. Family Meals: Involve your baby in family mealtimes to model healthy eating habits.

Here are detailed complementary feeding recipes for between the ages of 8 to 12 months:

HEALTHY KHICHDI:

Ingredients:

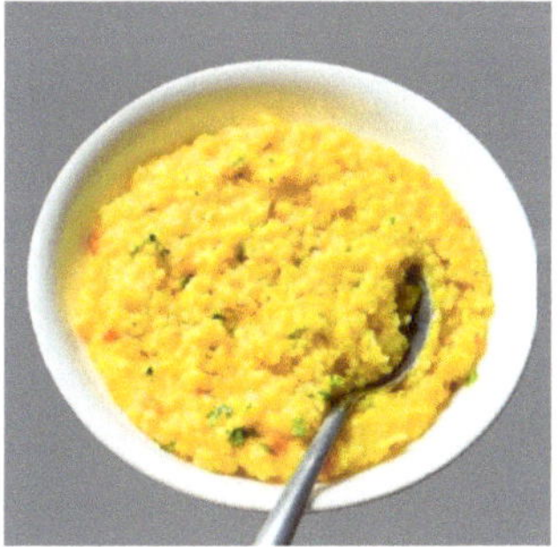

- 2/3 cup rice
- 1/3 cup Dal mix (1:1:1) = moong dal (yellow split lentils) + masoor dal (red lentils) + toor dal (pigeon peas)
- A pinch of turmeric powder
- 3 cups of water
- Ghee (optional)

Instructions:

- Wash all the lentils and rice thoroughly and soak them for about 30 minutes.
- In a pressure cooker, add the soaked lentils and rice along with a pinch of turmeric.
- Add 3 cups of water and pressure cook until you hear 3 whistles.
- Let the pressure release naturally, then open the lid and mash the khichdi to a soft consistency.
- You can add a teaspoon of ghee for added flavor and nutrition.

This khichdi will be rich in protein due to the variety of lentils used. You can also add finely chopped and cooked vegetables like spinach, carrots, or peas to increase the nutritional value.

BEETROOT RICE:

Ingredients:

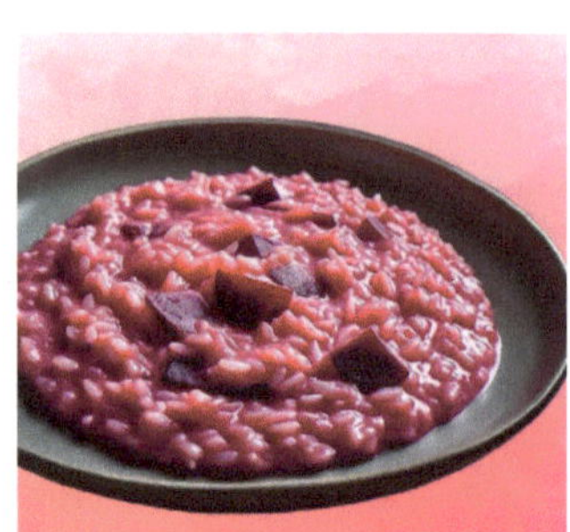

- 1/2 cup rice
- 1/4 cup grated beetroot
- 1/4 cup moong dal (split green gram)
- A pinch of turmeric powder
- Water (as needed for cooking)

Instructions:

- Wash the rice and moong dal thoroughly.
- In a pressure cooker, combine rice, grated beetroot, and moong dal.
- Add a pinch of turmeric powder and water (approximately 2 cups).
- Cook until it's soft and well-cooked.
- Mash or blend the mixture to the desired consistency.
- Serve warm to your little one.

LENTIL SOUP RECIPE WITH SPINACH (PALAK DAL):

Ingredients:

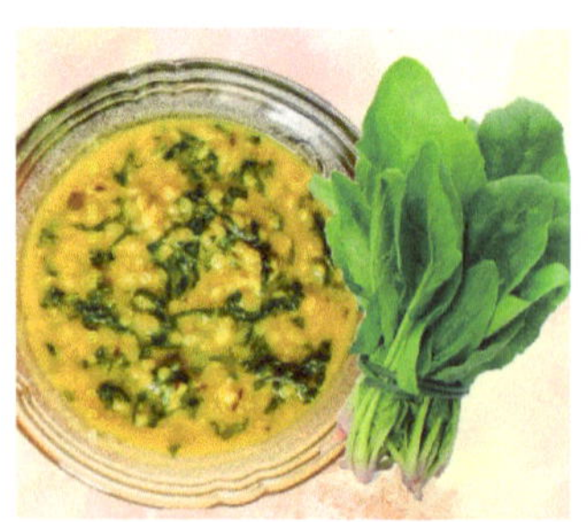

- 1/2 cup red lentils, washed and drained
- 1 small onion, finely chopped
- 1 carrot, peeled and diced
- 1 tomato, diced

- A handful of fresh spinach leaves, washed and chopped
- 2 cups vegetable broth or water
- A pinch of salt (optional, consult your pediatrician)
- Olive oil for cooking

Instructions:

- In a pot, heat a little olive oil and sauté the onion until translucent.
- Add the diced carrot and tomato to the pot and cook for a few minutes.
- Add the red lentils and vegetable broth or water. Bring to a boil, then reduce the heat and simmer until the lentils are soft, about 30 minutes.
- A few minutes before the soup is done, add the chopped spinach leaves and let them wilt in the hot soup.
- Once cooked, blend the soup to a smooth consistency or leave it chunky based on your baby's preference and feeding stage.

This soup is rich in protein from the lentils and vitamins from the vegetables, making it a wholesome meal for your baby. Always ensure the ingredients are soft enough for your baby to eat safely.

BROKEN WHEAT (DALIA) PORRIDGE WITH APPLES AND BANANAS:

Ingredients:

- 1/2 cup broken wheat (dalia/ godumai rava)
- 1 ripe banana
- 1 apple

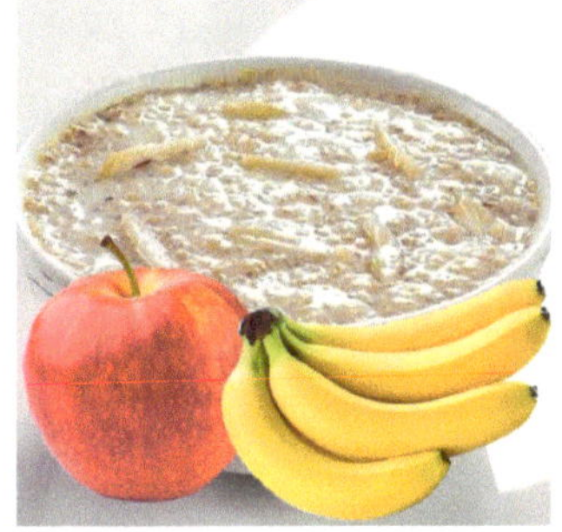

Instructions:

- Pressure cook the broken wheat with 1/2 cup water until soft.
- Peel and mash the banana finely.
- Peel, core, and chop the apple into small pieces.
- Boil the apple pieces in water until soft.
- Mash the cooked broken wheat, banana, and apple together.
- Serve this wholesome porridge to babies

RICE ALMOND DATES KHEER RECIPE:

Ingredients:

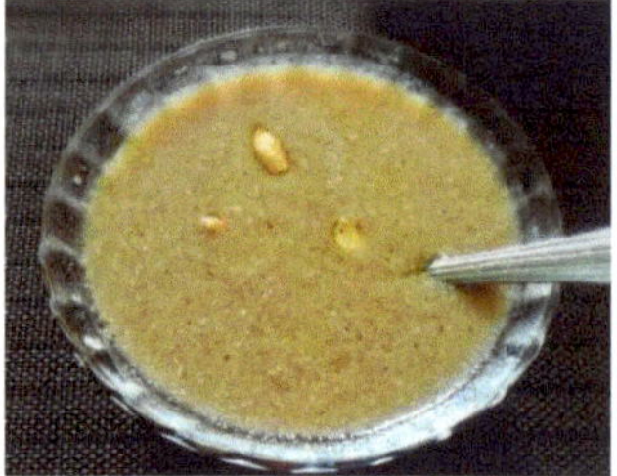

- 2 tablespoons rice
- 10 almonds (soaked and peeled)
- 5 dates (soaked and deseeded)
- 2 cups milk
- A pinch of saffron strands (optional)
- Chopped nuts (cashews, pistachios) for garnish

Instructions:

- Prepare the Rice Paste:
- Soak 2 tablespoons of rice in water for about 10-15 minutes.
- Drain and grind the rice to a smooth paste using a little water.
- Make Almond-Date Puree:
- Blend-soaked almonds and dates to a fine puree using a little water.

- Cook the Kheer:
- Boil 2 cups of milk in a heavy-bottomed pan.
- Add the rice paste, keeping the heat on medium/low.
- Stir continuously to avoid lumps.
- Once the rice is cooked and the kheer thickens, add the almond-date puree.
- Add saffron strands (if using). Mix well.
- Serve warm

Note: Adjust the sweetness (with dates) according to your child's preference.

These recipes provide essential nutrients and are gentle on the tummy. Enjoy!

<u>VEGETABLE IDLIS:</u>

Ingredients:

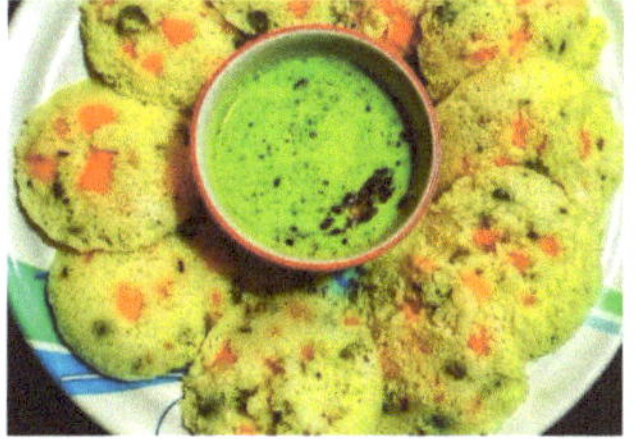

- 2 cups idli batter
- 1/2 cup finely chopped mixed vegetables (carrots, beans, peas, capsicum, etc.)
- 1/4 teaspoon turmeric powder (optional for color)
- Salt to taste
- Oil for greasing

Instructions:

- Prepare the idli batter as you normally would and let it ferment.
- Once the batter is fermented, add salt to taste and turmeric powder if using, and mix well.

- Heat a little oil in a pan and sauté the finely chopped vegetables with a pinch of salt for about 2-3 minutes until they are slightly soft. Allow them to cool.
- Mix the sautéed vegetables into the batter.
- Grease the idli molds with a little oil to prevent sticking.
- Pour the vegetable-laden batter into the greased idli molds.
- Steam the idlis in an idli steamer or pressure cooker (without the weight) for about 10-12 minutes. Check if they're done by inserting a toothpick; if it comes out clean, they're ready.
- Allow the idlis to cool for a couple of minutes before gently removing them from the molds.
- Serve the warm vegetable idlis with coconut chutney.

Enjoy this healthy and colorful meal with your little one!

<u>VEGETABLE SUJI:</u>

Ingredients:

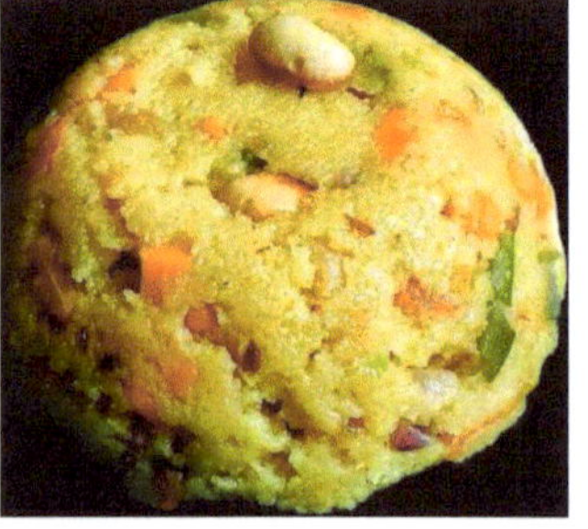

- 1/2 cup suji (semolina)
- 1/4 cup finely chopped onions
- 1/4 cup finely chopped tomatoes
- 1/4 cup finely chopped mixed vegetables (carrots, peas, beans)
- 1 tbsp ghee
- 1/2 tsp cumin seeds (jeera)
- A pinch of turmeric powder (haldi)
- Salt to taste
- Water as needed

Instructions:

- Heat ghee in a pan, add cumin seeds and let them crackle.
- Add onions and sauté until they turn slightly brown.
- Add tomatoes and cook until they become mushy.
- Add the mixed vegetables and turmeric powder, sauté for a minute.
- Add suji to the pan and roast it on a low flame until it turns light brown.Pour water gradually, stirring continuously to avoid lumps.
- Add salt, cover the pan, and cook on a low flame until the suji is cooked and the water is absorbed.
- Serve warm.

This dish is easy to digest and provides a good mix of carbohydrates, vitamins, and minerals.

Chapter 15

Toddlers Tasty Tales

1-2 years of wholesome meals

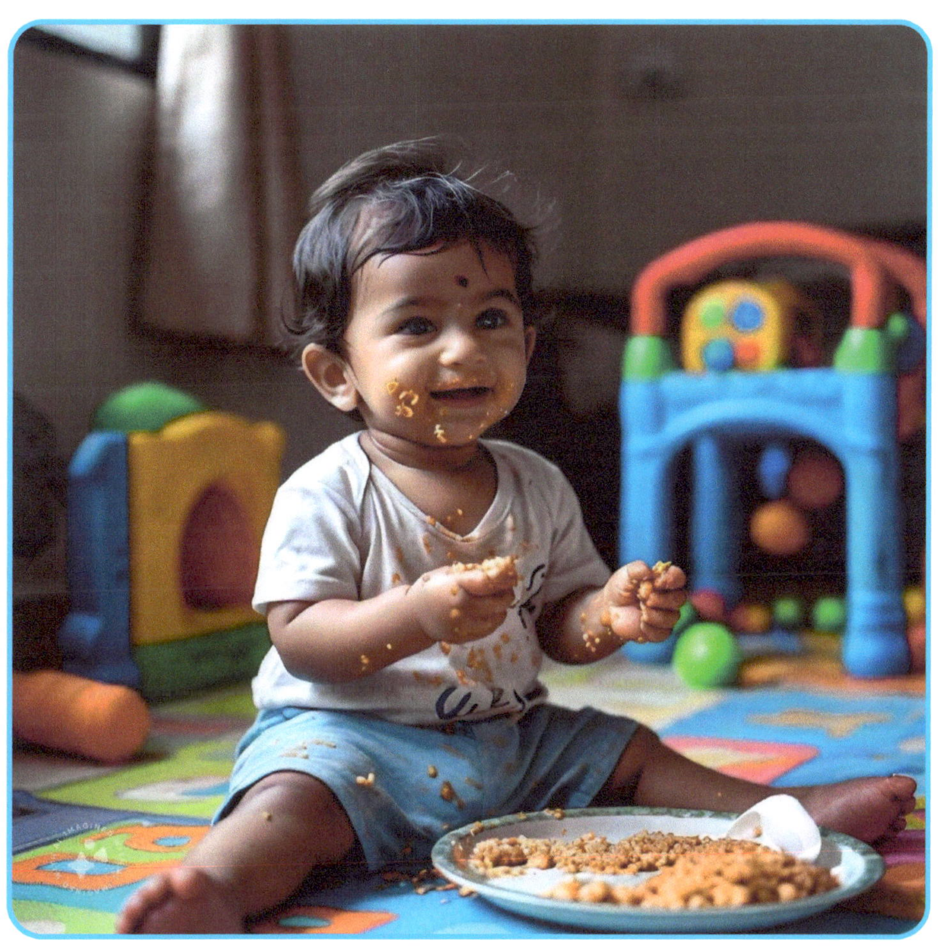

"Healthy food, healthy mind, healthy body - a bright future ahead."

"A healthy plate is a reflection of our love and care for our children's well-being."

– Dr. Nadia Shakoor

From 1 to 2 years, your child's developmental milestones continue to evolve, and their dietary needs grow. Here's how to support their readiness for more advanced complementary feeding:

Signs of Readiness:

1. Increased Coordination: Better control of utensils, such as a spoon and fork.

2. Greater Independence: Strong desire to self-feed and make choices about what to eat.

3. Complex Chewing and Swallowing: Ability to handle more complex food textures and larger pieces.

Benefits:

1. Autonomy and Confidence: Encouraging self-feeding fosters independence and self-confidence.

2. Nutritional Adequacy: Introducing a variety of foods ensures a balanced diet and meets nutritional needs.

3. Taste Development: Exposure to different flavors helps develop taste preferences and healthy eating habits.

Feeding Tips:

1. Offer Balanced Meals: Provide a variety of foods from all food groups to ensure balanced nutrition.

2. Let Them Choose: Allow your child to choose from healthy options to foster independence.

3. Family Meals: Continue involving your child in family meals.

Here are detailed complementary feeding recipes for between the ages of 1 to 2 years:

HOMEMADE POHA CEREAL MIX:

Ingredients:

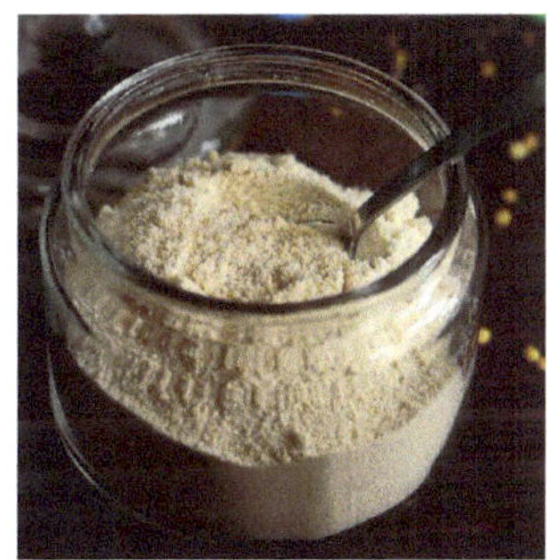

- 1 cup thick poha (beaten rice)
- ¼ cup roasted gram dal
- ⅛ cup almonds
- ⅛ cup cashews
- 1 green cardamom

Instructions:

- Dry roast the poha in a pan over low flame for 3-5 minutes until it becomes crispy and aromatic. Remove from the pan.
- In the same pan, dry roast the roasted gram dal until it's hot to touch. Remove from the pan.
- Roast the almonds, cashews, and green cardamom together for a minute. Switch off the flame.
- Grind the roasted poha into a smooth powder using a blender or mixer. Transfer it to a plate and let it cool.
- Next, grind the roasted gram dal into a smooth powder.
- Finally, blend the roasted nuts until well combined.
- Mix all the powdered ingredients together thoroughly.
- Store the homemade poha cereal mix in an airtight container.

<u>MILK POHA PORRIDGE (using homemade poha cereal mix):</u>

Ingredients:

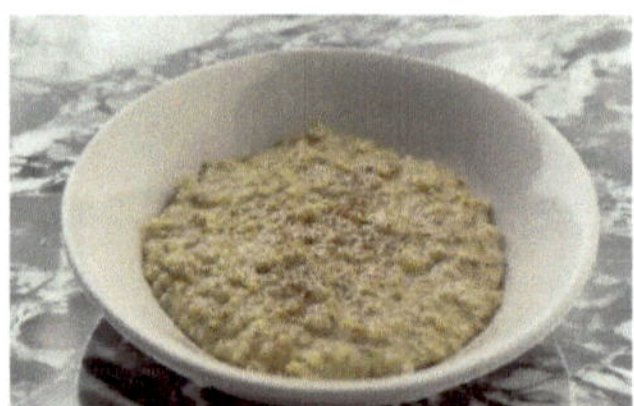

- 2 tablespoons homemade Poha Cereal Mix (see below for details)
- ¾ cup water
- 1-2 tablespoons jaggery (optional, adjust to taste)
- A pinch of salt (optional)
- ½ teaspoon ghee

Instructions:

- Heat jaggery in a pan with water until it reaches a slight honey-like consistency. Strain the jaggery water to remove impurities (optional).
- Take 2 tablespoons of poha cereal mix in a saucepan.
- Add ¾ cup of water and whisk well to ensure there are no lumps.
- Cook the porridge for 5 minutes until it thickens slightly.
- Add ghee and jaggery syrup (or salt) at this stage. Give it a quick stir.
- Cook for an additional 2 minutes and then switch off the flame.
- Cool the porridge and serve it warm.

Notes:

- Adjust the consistency by adding boiled water/formula or breast milk if the porridge becomes too thick.
- For toddlers above one year, you can use ¾ cup of boiled cow's milk instead of water.

- Skip jaggery or salt for babies below one year; use dates or raisins paste instead.

SPROUTED MOONG DAL DOSA RECIPE:

Ingredients:

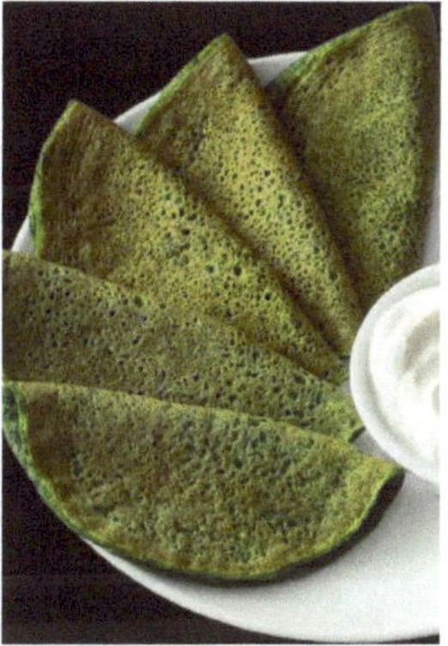

- 1 cup sprouted moong dal
- 1/4 cup rice flour (for crispiness, optional)
- 1/4 tsp cumin powder
- A pinch of asafoetida (hing)
- Salt to taste
- Water, as needed to make batter
- Ghee or oil, for cooking

Instructions:

- Grind the sprouted moong dal with a little water to make a smooth paste.
- Transfer the paste to a mixing bowl and add rice flour, cumin powder, asafoetida, and salt.
- Add water gradually to make a batter of pouring consistency.
- Heat a non-stick tawa (griddle) over medium-heat and grease it lightly with ghee or oil.
- Pour a ladleful of batter onto the tawa and spread it evenly to form a thin circle.
- Cook until the dosa is golden brown on one side, then flip and cook the other side.
- Serve warm with chutney or sauce of your choice.

This dosa is soft, nutritious, and perfect for your toddler's delicate palate.

<u>VEGETABLE PARATHA:</u>

Ingredients:

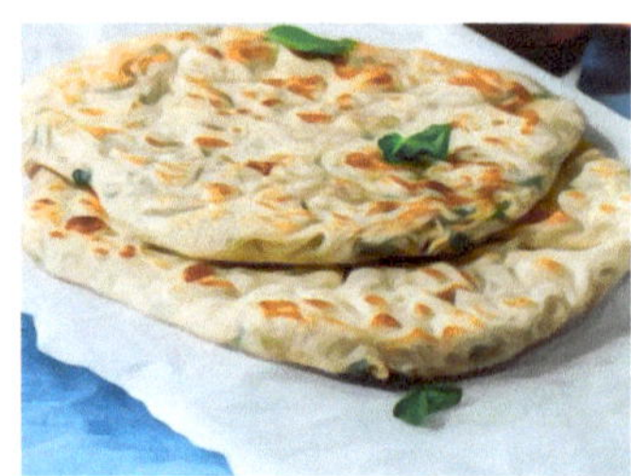

- 1 cup whole wheat flour
- Water as needed to make dough
- Salt to taste
- 1 cup mixed vegetables (carrots, cauliflower, peas, potatoes, beans), boiled and mashed
- Spices as per choice (pepper, coriander powder, etc.)
- Oil or ghee for cooking

Instructions:

- In a large bowl, mix the whole wheat flour and salt. Gradually add water and knead to form a soft dough. Set aside for 15-20 minutes.
- In another bowl, mix the mashed vegetables with your choice of spices.
- Divide the dough into small balls. Roll one ball into a small circle, place some vegetable mixture in the center, and seal it by bringing the edges together.
- Flatten the stuffed ball and roll it gently into a paratha of desired thickness.
- Heat a tawa or skillet and cook the paratha on both sides, applying oil or ghee until golden brown spots appear.
- Serve warm with yogurt or a mild chutney.

This vegetable paratha is not only nutritious but also a colorful way to include various vegetables in your child's diet.

<u>SUJI HALWA RECIPE USING DATES INSTEAD OF SUGAR:</u>

Ingredients:

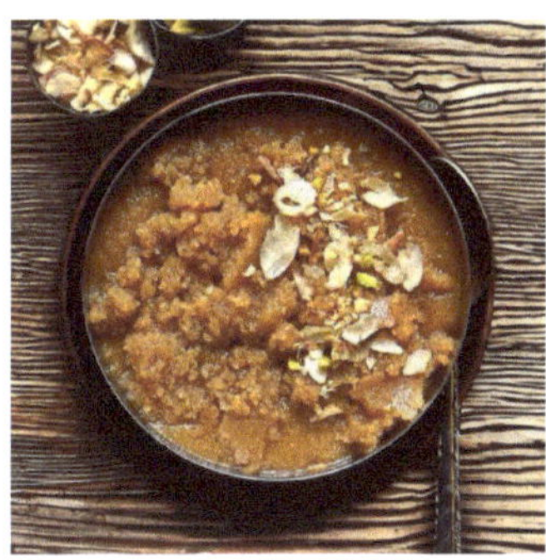

- 1 cup suji (semolina)
- 1/2 cup dates, pitted and chopped
- 1/4 cup ghee (clarified butter)
- 2 cups water
- 1/4 tsp cardamom powder
- Nuts and dried fruits for garnishing (optional)

Instructions:

- Soak the chopped dates in warm water for about 30 minutes to soften them.
- In a pan, heat the ghee over medium flame.
- Add the suji and roast it, stirring continuously until it turns golden brown and aromatic.
- Blend the soaked dates with a little water to make a smooth paste.
- Add the date paste to the roasted suji along with cardamom powder.
- Gradually add water while stirring continuously to avoid lumps.
- Cook until the mixture thickens and ghee starts separating from the sides of the pan.
- Garnish with nuts and dried fruits if desired.
- Serve warm.

This halwa is naturally sweetened with dates, making it a healthier option for your toddler.

PANEER DOSA RECIPE:

Ingredients:

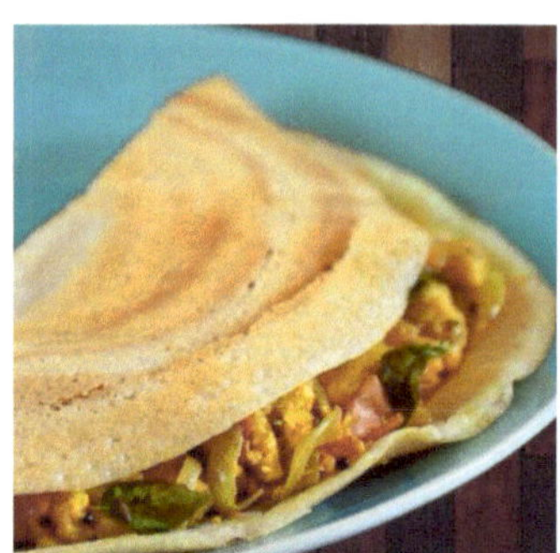

- 1 cup dosa batter (ready-made or homemade)
- 200g paneer (cottage cheese), crumbled
- 1/4 cup capsicum, finely chopped
- 1/4 cup onion, finely chopped (optional)
- 1/4 tsp turmeric powder
- Salt to taste
- Oil, for cooking

Instructions:

- In a bowl, mix crumbled paneer, capsicum, onion (if using), turmeric powder, and salt.
- Heat a non-stick tawa (griddle) over medium-heat and grease it lightly with oil.
- Pour a ladleful of dosa batter onto the tawa and spread it evenly to form a thin circle.
- Place a portion of the paneer mixture on one half of the dosa.
- Drizzle some oil around the edges and cook until the dosa is golden brown and crispy.
- Fold the dosa over the filling and remove from tawa.
- Serve warm with coconut chutney or tomato sauce.

This paneer dosa is a great way to add protein to your toddler's diet and can be enjoyed as a wholesome breakfast or snack.

<u>VEGETABLE EGG OMELET RECIPE:</u>

Ingredients:

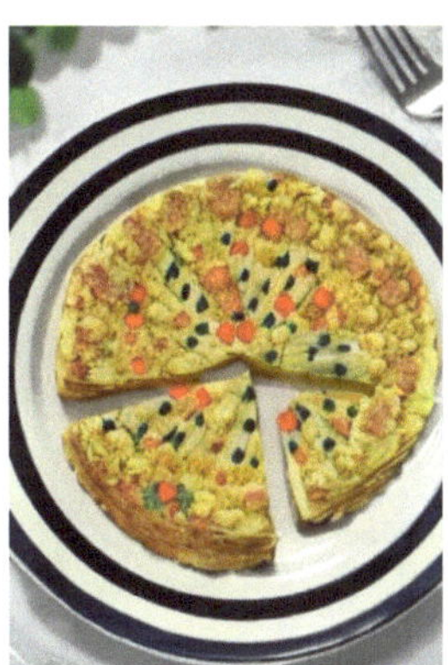

- 2 eggs
- 1 tbsp milk (optional, for fluffiness)
- 1/4 cup finely chopped vegetables (capsicum, tomatoes, onions, spinach)
- A pinch of turmeric powder (optional, for color)
- A pinch of black pepper (optional)
- Cheese (optional, for added taste and calcium)
- 1 tsp butter or oil

Instructions:

- In a bowl, whisk the eggs with milk, turmeric, and black pepper until well combined.
- Stir in the finely chopped vegetables.
- Heat butter or oil in a non-stick pan over medium-heat.
- Pour the egg mixture into the pan.
- Cook until the edges start to lift from the pan, then gently flip the omelet to cook the other side.
- If using cheese, sprinkle it on top and fold the omelet in half.
- Cook for another minute until the cheese is melted and the omelet is cooked through.
- Serve warm.

This omelet is packed with protein and veggies, making it a wholesome meal for your little one.

VEGETABLE PANCAKE:

Ingredients:

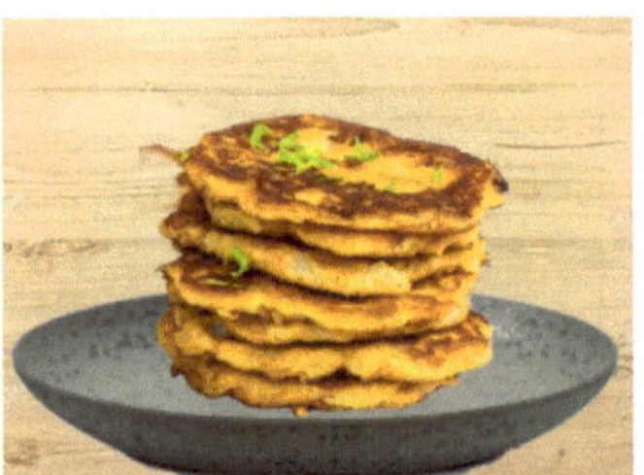

- 1/2 cup rice flour
- 1/2 cup chickpea flour (besan)
- 1/4 cup finely chopped mixed vegetables (carrots, bell peppers, spinach)
- 1/4 tsp baking powder
- A pinch of salt
- Water, as needed to make a thick batter
- Oil, for cooking

Instructions:

- In a bowl, mix together rice flour, chickpea flour, baking powder, and salt.
- Gradually add water to make a thick batter.
- Stir in the finely chopped vegetables.
- Let the batter rest for 10 minutes.
- Heat a non-stick pan over medium-heat and brush with oil.
- Pour spoonfuls of batter onto the pan to form small pancakes.
- Cook until the edges are set and the bottom is golden brown, then flip and cook the other side.
- Serve warm.

These pancakes are a great way to include a variety of vegetables in your toddler's diet and can be served with a yogurt dip.

<u>GHEE CHICKEN RICE:</u>

Ingredients:

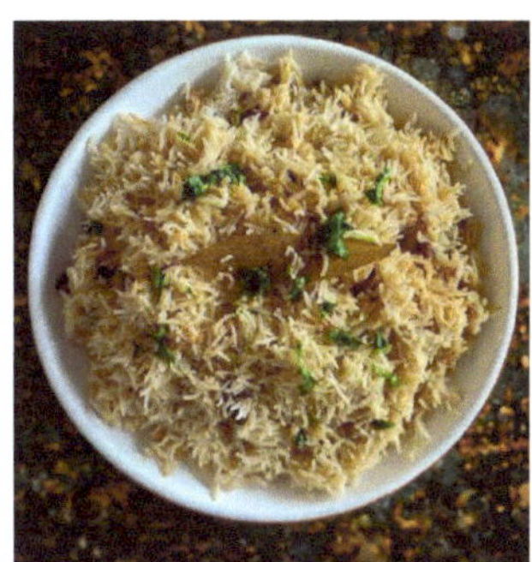

- 1 cup cooked rice (preferably brown rice for added fiber)
- 1 boneless chicken breast, cooked and shredded
- 1/4 cup cooked and finely chopped carrots
- 1/4 cup cooked and finely chopped peas
- 1/4 cup cooked and finely chopped broccoli
- 1/2 cup whole milk or unsweetened yogurt
- 1 tablespoon ghee
- A pinch of black pepper (optional)

Instructions:

- In a saucepan, ghee over low-heat.
- Add the shredded chicken and sauté for a minute.
- Add the cooked rice, carrots, peas, and broccoli. Mix well.
- Pour in the milk or yogurt and stir until everything is combined.
- Season with a pinch of black pepper if desired.
- Serve warm to your little one!

Remember to cut the chicken and veggies into toddler-friendly sizes.

This dish provides a good balance of protein, carbohydrates, and veggies, making it a wholesome meal for growing toddlers.

SPROUTS FRANKIE RECIPE:

Ingredients:

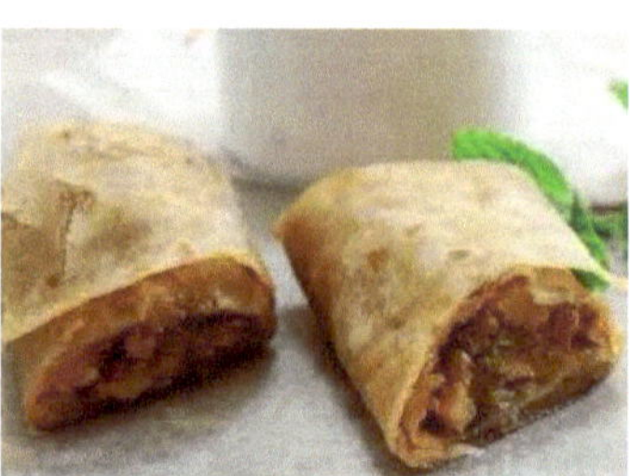

- 1 whole wheat tortilla or chapati (roti)
- 1/2 cup mixed sprouts (such as mung bean sprouts, lentil sprouts, or chickpea sprouts)
- 1/4 cup finely chopped bell peppers (red, green, or yellow)
- 1/4 cup grated carrot
- 1/4 cup finely chopped cucumber
- 1/4 cup cooked and mashed sweet potato
- 1/4 teaspoon cumin powder
- A pinch of black salt (kala namak) for flavor
- 1 teaspoon ghee or oil for cooking

Instructions:

- Heat the ghee or oil in a pan.
- Add the mixed sprouts and sauté for a few minutes until they are slightly tender.
- Sprinkle cumin powder and black salt over the sprouts and mix well.
- Warm the whole wheat tortilla or chapati on a griddle.
- Spread the mashed sweet potato evenly on the tortilla.
- Arrange the sautéed sprouts, chopped bell peppers, grated carrot, and cucumber on top.
- Roll up the tortilla tightly to form a frankie.
- Cut the frankie into toddler-friendly pieces.

Serve this wholesome and colorful sprouts frankie to your little one!

It's packed with fiber, vitamins, and protein. Enjoy!

EGG PARATHA (ANDA PARATHA):

Ingredients:

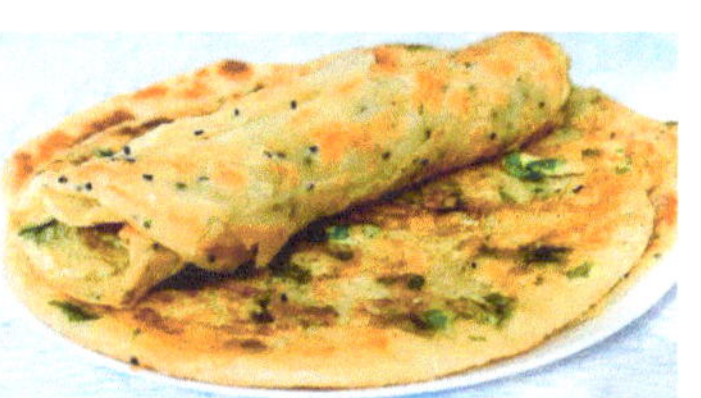

- 1 cup whole wheat flour (atta)
- Salt, to taste
- Water, as needed
- 2 eggs
- 1 small onion, finely chopped
- 1 green chili, finely chopped (optional; adjust for kids)
- A handful of fresh coriander leaves, chopped
- Oil or ghee for cooking

Instructions:

- Prepare the Dough:
- In a mixing bowl, add half a cup of wheat flour and a pinch of salt.
- Gradually pour in warm water (about 3 tablespoons) and knead to form a soft, non-sticky dough. Add more water if needed.
- Smear a few drops of oil on the dough, cover, and set it aside.
- Prepare the Egg Mixture:
- Whisk together 2 eggs, chopped onion, green chili (if using), and coriander leaves. Set aside.
- Roll the Parathas:
- Divide the dough into 2 equal portions and roll them into smooth balls.
- Flour the rolling surface lightly and coat the balls with flour on both sides.
- Roll each ball into a round 6-inch roti.

- Layered Paratha (Optional):
- Apply ¼ teaspoon of oil all over the rolled-out roti.
- Fold it in half to form a pocket.
- Roll it again into a circle of 6 inches.
- Cook the Paratha:
- Heat a non-stick tava (griddle) and grease it with 1 teaspoon of oil or ghee.
- Pour half of the egg mixture onto the tava.
- Place a prepared paratha on top and press it lightly.
- Cook until the egg is set.
- Flip the paratha and cook the other side until fully cooked.

"Teach your child to eat a rainbow, and they'll be eating a rainbow of nutrients."

In conclusion, a nutritious meal is a big hug for a child's body and soul, setting them up for a bright future. Healthy children, happy parents - the circle of nutrition is a vital one, where balanced diets and happy hearts go hand in hand. By providing our children with the building blocks of nutritious food, we watch them grow into strong, confident individuals, equipped to take on the world.

Let us cherish the power of nutrition and nurture our children's bodies and souls, setting them up for a lifetime of health, happiness, and success.

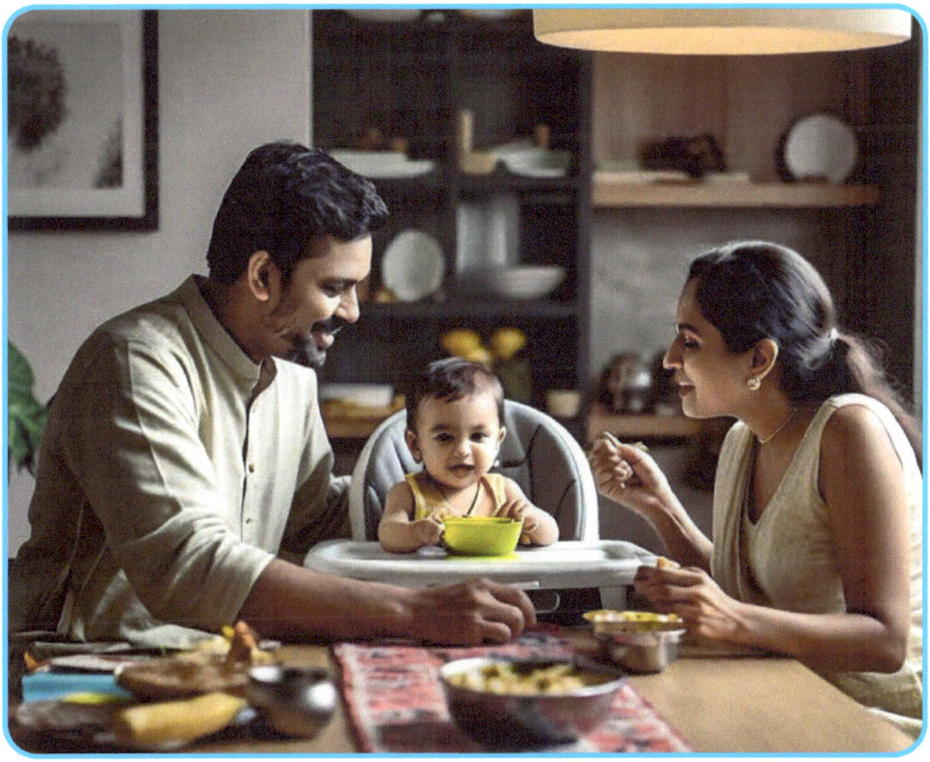

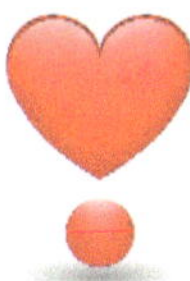

HAPPY PARENTING

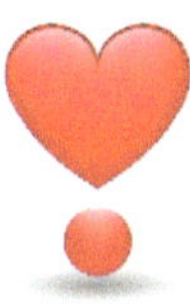

www.ingramcontent.com/pod-product-compliance
Lightning Source LLC
Chambersburg PA
CBHW040853110726
48005CB00001B/42